CLINICAL PHARMACOLOGY MADE RIDICULOUSLY SIMPLE

6th Edition

James M. Olson, M.D., Ph.D.

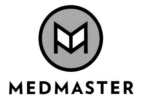

MEDMASTER

Clinical Pharmacology Made Ridiculously Simple aims at providing general principles of pharmacology and is not intended as a working guide to patient drug administration. Please refer to the manufacturer's package insert for recommended drug dosage, undesirable effects, contraindications and drug interactions.

ISBN 9781935660705
eISBN 9781935660712

Made in the United States of America

Published by
MedMaster, Inc.
P.O. Box 640028
Miami, FL 33164

For Rose Olson

SPECIAL THANKS TO:

THE ILLUSTRATORS
Deb Haimes
Josh Worth
Matteo Farinella
Nancy Ciliax
Isabel Loureiro

THE BOOK REVIEWERS
Jang-Ho Cha, M.D., Ph.D.
Stephen Goldberg, M.D.
Jorge Iñiguez-Lluhí, Ph.D.
Joanne Finnorn, J.D.

THE CHAPTER AND TABLE REVIEWERS/CONTRIBUTORS
Rosemary Berardi, Pharm. D.
Anne Bournay, R.Ph.
Kevin Cassady, M.D.
Betty Chaffee, Pharm. D.
Tim Esser, M.D.
Marc Fischer, M.D.
Janet Gilsdorf, M.D.
Eric Hockstad, M.D.
Roy Kulick, M.D.
Jorge Iñiguez-Lluhí, Ph.D.
Fred Lamb, M.D., Ph.D.
Lori Mangels, Ph.D.
Beverly Mitchell, M.D.
Charles Neal, M.D., Ph.D.
Francis Pasely, M.D.
John Penney, M.D.
Anna Porcari, Pharm. D.
Rudy Roskos, M.D.
Anne Ruch, M.D.
Raymond Ruddon, M.D., Ph.D.
Steve Silverman, M.D.
Helen Yun, Pharm. D., M.B.A.

Contents

Preface

I developed the format of this book while teaching a review course in pharmacology to medical students who were having difficulty with the standard course. The students stated that the concepts of pharmacology were not difficult, but that they were overwhelmed by the quantity of material. They spent hours leafing through pages, trying to identify subtle differences between drugs that have similar names, actions, pharmacokinetics and side effects.

This guide organizes related drugs in tables. It allows the student to learn about a prototype drug and the important ways that related drugs differ. The text that surrounds the tables emphasizes key issues pertaining to therapeutic rationale, basic pharmacologic principles and clinical use of the drugs.

The book blends the essentials of basic pharmacology and clinical pharmacology so that the transition from classroom to clinical setting is less abrupt. Students report that the book is most effective when lecture notes are written directly on the tables and margins, providing a single, concise guide for finals and the Boards. The book can then be used during clinical training for a rapid review of the principles that guide rational prescribing practices.

Clinical Pharmacology Made Ridiculously Simple contains the information required to perform well on the Boards and to answer most pharmacology questions asked during clinical rounds. It does not present historical aspects of pharmacology, exhaustive lists of side effects and drug interactions, or other details that are best found in traditional texts or formularies.

I welcome comments and suggestions for future editions.

Jim Olson, M.D., Ph.D.
Children's Hospital/University of Washington/Fred Hutchinson Cancer Center
1920 Terry Ave.
Seattle, WA 98101

Chapter 1 **Principles of Pharmacology**

Rational Therapeutics

There are thousands of drugs and hundreds of facts about each of them. It is unnecessary to memorize many of these facts if one learns to predict the behavior of each drug based on a few facts and an understanding of the principles of pharmacology.

This chapter presents the basic principles of pharmacology upon which drug therapy is based. As you read the chapter, try to apply the principles to a drug with which you are familiar. Refer to this chapter often as you learn the drugs presented in the rest of the book. Try to learn the "story" of each drug rather than isolated facts. The best way to develop a story about a drug is to **associate, ask, and predict.**

Associate each drug class with information that you already know about the drugs. Think of relatives or friends who have taken medicine from the class of drugs you are studying. Remember what you have read or heard about the drugs.

Ask yourself why some drugs are administered as shots and others as pills, why some drugs are taken four times daily and others only once, and why it is important for a health care provider to know the serum concentration of some drugs but not of others. As you read the following chapters, ask yourself "Why is this information important enough to be included in this book?".

Predict the actions, clinical uses, side effects, and drug interactions of each drug based solely on its mechanism of action. If you can predict these characteristics, you will only have to memorize those facts that do not make intuitive sense.

Finally, envision the course of events that would occur as a drug enters the patient's body. Continue this practice each time you prescribe, dispense or administer drugs to a patient. Your patients will benefit if your clinical decisions are determined rationally and based on a foundation of basic pharmacology knowledge.

Drug Administration

• *Formulation*

Clinically useful drugs are formulated by drug companies into preparations that can be administered orally, intravenously, or by another route. **The formulation of a drug depends on the following factors:**

- **The barriers that the drug is capable of passing.** Intravenous drugs are injected directly into the blood stream. In contrast, oral preparations must pass through the wall of the gastrointestinal tract and blood vessel walls before entering the bloodstream.

- **The setting in which the drug will be used.** An intravenous preparation might be appropriate for a drug which is administered during surgery, but would be inappropriate for home administration.

- **The urgency of the medical situation.** The delay before onset of action varies between preparations of the same drug. Emergency situations often call for intravenous administration of agents which might normally be administered by another route.
- **Stability of the drug.** Drugs which are denatured by acid are not good candidates for oral preparations because they may be destroyed in the stomach (stomach pH = 2).
- **First Pass Effect.** Blood from the gastrointestinal tract passes through the liver before entering any other organs. During this first pass through the liver, a fraction of the drug (in some cases nearly all) can be metabolized to an inactive or less active derivative. The inactivation of some drugs is so great that the agents are useless when administered orally.

• *Routes of Drug Administration*

Routes of drug administration include:

- **Oral (PO):** Most compatible with drugs that are self-administered. Oral agents must be able to withstand the acidic environment of the stomach and must permeate the gut lining before entering the blood-stream. Absorption affected by gastric emptying and intestinal motility.
- **Sublingual:** Good absorption through capillary bed under tongue. Drugs are easily self-administered. Because the stomach is bypassed, acid-lability and gut-permeability need not be considered.
- **Rectal (PR):** Useful for unconscious or vomiting patients or small children. Absorption is unreliable.
- **Inhalation:** Generally rapid absorption. Some agents, marketed in devices which deliver metered doses, are suitable for self-administration.
- **Topical:** Useful for local delivery of agents, particularly those which have toxic effects if administered systemically. Used for most dermatologic, ophthalmologic, nasal, vaginal, and otic preparations.
- **Transdermal:** A few drugs can be formulated such that a "patch" containing the drug is applied to the skin. The drug seeps out of the patch, through the skin and into the capillary bed. Very convenient for self-administration.

There are three drug administration techniques which have traditionally been labeled **parenteral** ("around the gastrointestinal tract"). Advantages include more rapid and predictable absorption and more accurate dose selection. Disadvantages include the need for strict asepsis, risk of infection, pain, and local irritation.

- **Intravenous (IV):** Rapid onset of action because agent is injected directly into the blood stream. Useful in emergencies and in patients that are unconscious. Insoluble drugs cannot be administered intravenously.
- **Intramuscular (IM):** Drug passes through capillary walls to enter the blood stream. Rate of absorption depends on formulation (oil-based preparations are absorbed slowly, aqueous preparations are absorbed rapidly). May be used for self-administration by trained patients.
- **Subcutaneous (SubQ, SC):** Drug is injected beneath the skin and permeates capillary walls to enter the blood stream. Absorption can be controlled by drug formulation. Only nonirritating drugs can be used.

• *Dosing Regimens*

Three common dosing regimens are compared in Table 1.1. The **half-life** is the amount of time required for the plasma concentration of a drug to decrease by 50% after discontinuance of the drug. The **distribution half-life** ($t_{1/2}\alpha$) reflects the rapid decline in plasma drug concentration as a dose of drug is distributed throughout the body. The **elimination half-life** ($t_{1/2}\beta$) is often much slower, reflecting the metabolism and excretion of the drug. Note that several half-lives pass before the serum concentration of a drug reaches steady state. Thus in order to obtain values which reflect the steady state, it is necessary to wait until the fourth or fifth half-life of a drug before the peak, trough or plasma level is measured.

Therapeutic levels of a drug can be obtained more rapidly by delivering a loading dose followed by maintenance doses. A **loading dose** is an initial dose of drug that is higher than subsequent doses for the purpose of achieving therapeutic drug concentrations in the serum rapidly. The loading dose is followed by **maintenance doses,** which are doses of drug that maintain a steady state plasma concentration in the therapeutic range.

The dosing regimen (route, amount, and frequency) of drug administration influences the onset and duration of drug action. **Onset** is the amount of time it takes a drug to begin working. Drugs administered intravenously generally have a more rapid onset than drugs taken orally because oral agents must be absorbed and pass through the gut before entering the bloodstream. **Duration** is the length of time for which a drug is therapeutic. The duration usually corresponds to the half-life of the drug (except when the drug binds irreversibly to its receptor) and is dependent on metabolism and excretion of the drug.

Table 1.1 Influence of Dosing Regimen on Plasma Drug Levels

DOSING REGIMEN	GRAPH OF PLASMA DRUG CONCENTRATION
Single Dose Plasma concentration of drug rises as the drug distributes to the bloodstream, then falls as the drug is distributed to tissues, metabolized, and excreted. Drugs administered orally reach a peak plasma concentration at a later time than drugs administered intravenously. Oral agents must be absorbed across GI mucosa and capillary walls before entering the bloodstream.	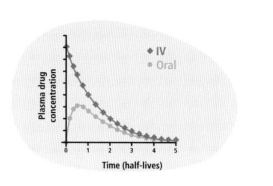
Continuous Infusion (IV) Steady state (equilibrium) plasma drug concentration is reached after continuous infusion for 4-5 half-lives. Increasing the rate of infusion will not decrease the time needed to reach steady state. Increasing the rate of infusion will, however, increase the plasma drug concentration at steady state.	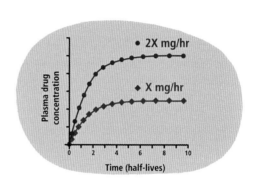
Intermittent Dose A drug must be administered for 4-5 half-lives before steady state (equilibrium) is reached. **Peaks** are the high points of fluctuation. Toxic effects may be caused by peak drug concentrations. **Troughs** are the low points of fluctuation. Lack of drug effect is most likely to occur during troughs. For example, post-operative pain is more likely to return just before a second dose of morphine than midway between the first and second dose.	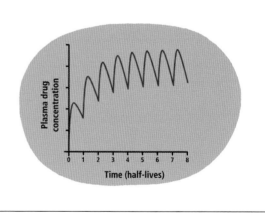

Pharmacokinetics

• Drug Absorption

As a drug is distributed in the body, it comes in contact with numerous membranes. Drugs pass some membranes but not others. Table 1.2 compares four drug transport mechanisms.

- **Drug-associated factors** that influence absorption include ionization state, molecular weight, solubility (lipophilicity) and formulation (solution vs. tablet). Small, nonionized, lipid-soluble drugs permeate plasma membranes most readily.

- **Patient-associated factors** that influence drug absorption depend on the route of administration. For example, the presence of food in the GI tract, stomach acidity and blood flow to the GI tract influence the absorption of oral medications.

Table 1.2 Drug Transport Across Membranes

MECHANISM	ENERGY	CARRIER	NOTES
Passive Diffusion	No	No	Rapid for lipophilic, nonionic and small molecules. Slow for hydrophilic, ionic, or large molecules.
Facilitated Diffusion	No	Yes	Drugs bind to carrier by noncovalent mechanisms. Chemically similar drugs compete for carrier.
Aqueous Channels	No	No	Small hydrophilic drugs (<200 mw) diffuse along concentration gradient by passing through aqueous channels (pores).
Active Transport	Yes	Yes	Identical to facilitated diffusion except that ATP powers drug transport against concentration gradient.

• *Drug Distribution*

The following factors influence drug distribution:

- **Membrane permeability:** In order to enter an organ, a drug must permeate all membranes that separate the organ from the site of drug administration. For example, benzodiazepines, which are very lipophilic, readily cross the gut wall, capillary wall, and **blood-brain barrier.** Because of this, they distribute to the brain rapidly and are useful for treating anxiety and seizures. In contrast, some antibiotics are capable of passing from the gut into the blood stream, but cannot pass into the brain. These drugs cannot be used to treat infections in the brain. Poor passage of some anticancer agents across the blood-brain barrier and the **blood-testes barrier** results in relatively high rates of brain or testicular recurrences of some tumors. The **blood-placenta barrier** prevents fetal exposure to some drugs but allows passage of others.

- **Plasma protein binding** (Fig. 1.1)**:** The binding of drugs to plasma proteins, such as albumin, reduces the amount of "free" (that which is not protein bound) drug in the blood. "Free" drug molecules, but not protein-bound molecules, reach an equilibrium between the blood and tissues. Thus a decrease in free drug in the serum translates to a decrease in drug which can enter a given organ.

- **Depot storage: Lipophilic drugs,** such as the sedative thiopental, accumulate in fat. These agents are released slowly from the fat stores. Thus, an obese person might be sedated for a greater period of time than a lean person to whom the same dose of thiopental had been administered. **Calcium-binding**

drugs, such as the antibiotic tetracycline, accumulate in bone and teeth.

The **apparent volume of distribution (V_d)** is a *calculated value* that describes the nature of drug distribution. V_d is *the volume that would be required to contain the administered dose if that dose was evenly distributed at the concentration measured in plasma.* You could predict that a drug with $V_d = 3$ liters is distributed in plasma only (plasma volume = 3 liters), whereas a drug with $V_d = 16$ liters is likely distributed in extracellular water (extracellular water = 3 liters plasma plus 10-13 liters interstitial fluid). A drug with $V_d > 46$ liters is likely sequestered in a depot because the body only contains 40-46 liters of fluid.

• *Drug Metabolism*

Drugs, chemicals, and toxins are all foreign to our bodies. Our body attempts to rid itself of foreign chemicals, regardless of whether they are therapeutic or harmful. Most drugs must be biotransformed, or metabolized, before they can be excreted. In pharmacology, the word "metabolism" often refers to the process of making a drug more polar and water soluble. Although this often results in drug inactivation and excretion, it is INCORRECT to assume that a metabolite will be less active or more easily excreted than the parent drug.

Metabolic reactions can transform . . .
- an active drug into less-active or inactive forms.
- a PRODRUG (inactive or less-active drug) into a more active drug.

Drug and toxin metabolism is divided into "Phase I" and "Phase II" reactions (Figures 1.2A, 1.2B).

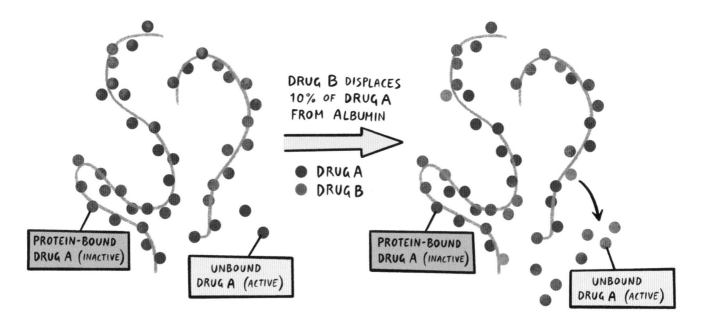

Figure 1.1 Consequence of drug displacement from albumin and other plasma proteins. Some drugs (e.g., "Drug A" in figure) are greater than 90% bound to plasma proteins. The "free" (unbound) drug molecules, but not the bound molecules, are available to act at receptors. In the figure, "Drug B" displaces only 5 molecules of "Drug A", which more than triples the serum concentration of free (active) "Drug A". This could be fatal if "Drug A" has a narrow margin of safety. Displacement of drugs which are less-highly protein bound is less significant. For example, if "Drug A" were 50% bound and 50% free, displacement of 10% of the bound fraction would increase the free fraction from 50% to 55%. This small increment is unlikely to be clinically relevant.

In Phase I Reactions (nonsynthetic), drugs are oxidized or reduced to a more polar form. In **Phase II Reactions (synthetic),** a polar group, such as glutathione, is conjugated to the drug. This substantially increases the polarity of the drug. Drugs undergoing Phase II conjugation reactions may have already undergone Phase I transformation.

The liver microsomal drug oxidation/reduction system (P450/CYP system) is responsible for the metabolism of many drugs. Cytochrome P450 (so named because it maximally absorbs light at 450 nm) is a family of isoenzymes located in the endoplasmic reticulum of the hepatocytes. Through an electron transport chain which uses NADPH as a proton carrier, a drug bound to cytochrome P450 can be oxidized or reduced (Phase I Reaction).

Cytochrome P450 can be *induced* (increased in activity) by a number of drugs or chemicals. Induction occurs in response to the presence of a chemical which is metabolized by P450 (more enzyme is produced to handle the chemical load). Once the enzyme is induced, it will metabolize the "inducing agent" more rapidly. Because cytochrome P450 is not specific for the inducer, however, other drugs metab-

olized by the *induced enzyme will also be biotransformed more rapidly.*

• *Drug Excretion*

Some drugs are excreted from the body after they have been metabolized to more polar congeners, while others are excreted "unchanged". Most drugs, toxins, and metabolites are excreted in the urine. Others are excreted in feces or expired air. Drugs that are excreted in the feces may be concentrated in bile before entering the intestine. In some cases, these drugs are reabsorbed into the portal bloodstream as they move through the intestines. This cycle, **enterohepatic circulation,** can extend the duration of the drug in the body.

A number of processes occur in the kidney which affect the rate of drug excretion. The most important processes are glomerular filtration, tubular secretion, and tubular reabsorption. These processes are compared in Table 1.3. Drug excretion mechanisms are vulnerable to renal insults such as toxins, other drugs, or disease states. Because drugs, metabolites, and toxins are concentrated in the kidney, the organ is

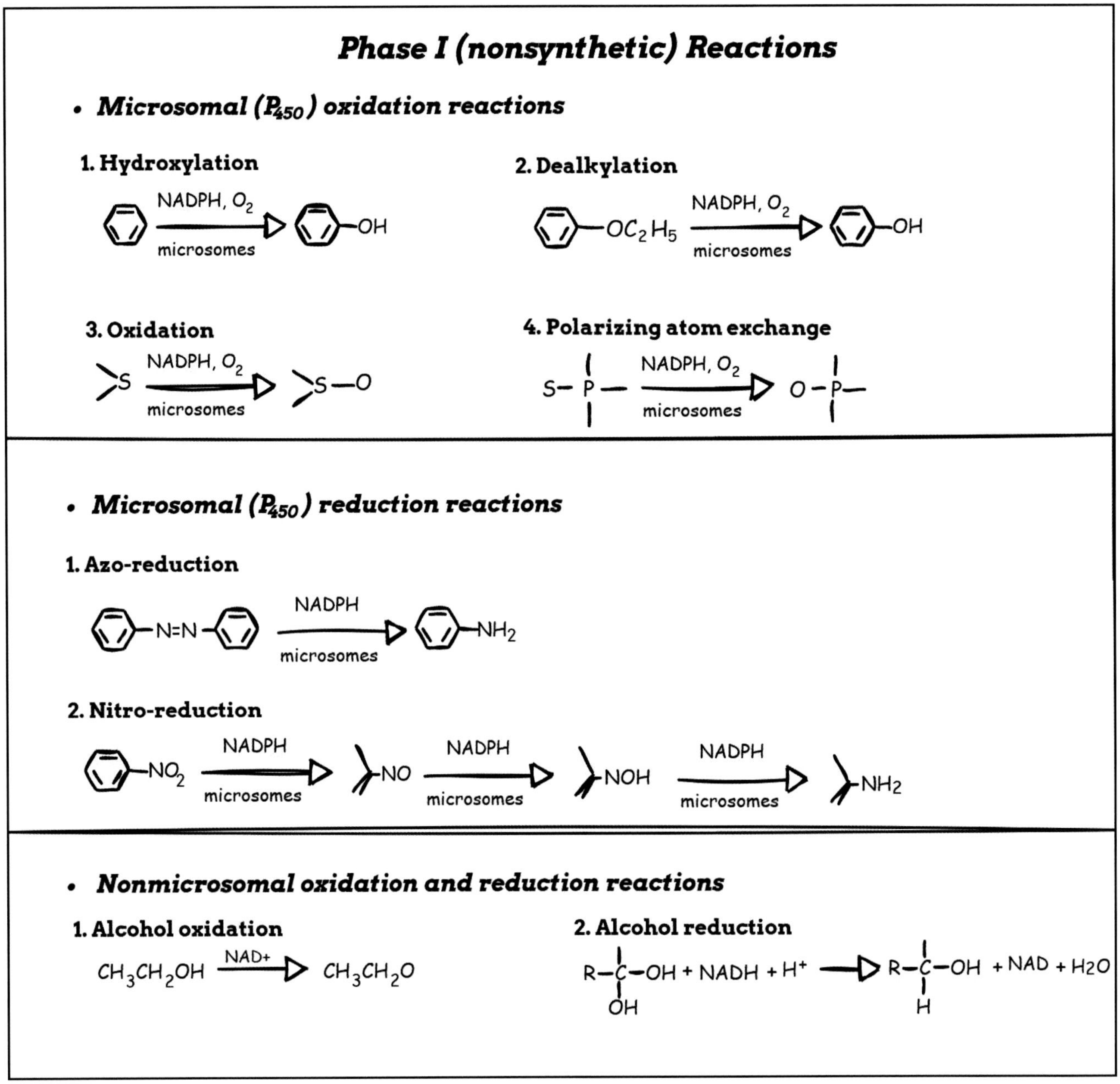

Phase I (nonsynthetic) Reactions
• Microsomal (P450) oxidation reactions
1. Hydroxylation
NADPH, O2
microsomes
OH
2. Dealkylation
OC2H5
NADPH, O2
microsomes
OH
3. Oxidation
S
NADPH, O2
microsomes
S—O
4. Polarizing atom exchange
S—P—
NADPH, O2
microsomes
O—P—
• Microsomal (P450) reduction reactions
1. Azo-reduction
N=N
NADPH
microsomes
NH2
2. Nitro-reduction
NO2
NADPH
microsomes
NO
NADPH
microsomes
NOH
NADPH
microsomes
NH2
• Nonmicrosomal oxidation and reduction reactions
1. Alcohol oxidation
CH3CH2OH
NAD+
CH3CH2O
2. Alcohol reduction
R—C—OH + NADH + H+
OH
R—C—OH + NAD + H2O
H

Figure 1.2A Examples of Phase I metabolic reactions.

frequently the site of chemical-induced toxicity. Undesirable symptoms in a patient with renal failure may be due to drug accumulation rather than the disease process itself.

• Drug Clearance

The term "clearance" refers to the volume of fluid that would be completely cleared of drug (per unit time) if all the drug being excreted/metabolized were removed from that volume (and the remaining fluid in the body retained the original concentration of drug). "Clearance" is a calculated value that cannot be directly measured in the body. It is measured in liters per hour, but is often mistaken for "rate of elimination" which is reported as mg/hr. Clearance values can be calculated for specific systems. For example, total clearance = renal clearance +

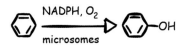

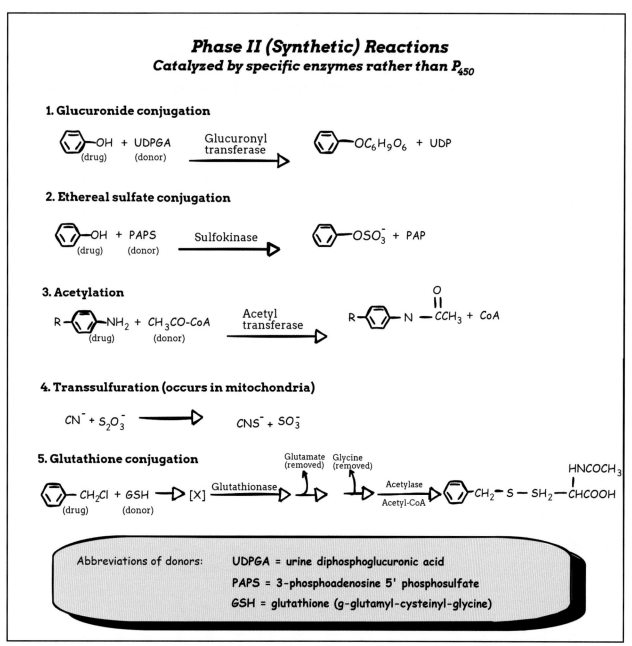

Phase II (Synthetic) Reactions
Catalyzed by specific enzymes rather than P_{450}

1. Glucuronide conjugation

2. Ethereal sulfate conjugation

3. Acetylation

4. Transsulfuration (occurs in mitochondria)

5. Glutathione conjugation

Abbreviations of donors:
UDPGA = urine diphosphoglucuronic acid
PAPS = 3-phosphoadenosine 5' phosphosulfate
GSH = glutathione (g-glutamyl-cysteinyl-glycine)

Figure 1.2B Examples of Phase II metabolic reactions.

metabolic clearance + all other clearance. Clearance can be calculated several ways:

$$\text{Clearance} = \frac{\text{Elimination Rate (mg/hr)}}{\text{Drug Concentration (mg/L)}} = \frac{\text{Liters}}{\text{hour}}$$

OR

$$\text{Clearance} = k \cdot V_d$$

Where k = elimination rate constant
and V_d = apparent volume of distribution

Drug Actions

Most drugs bind to cellular receptors, where they initiate a series of biochemical reactions that alter the cell's physiology. In a given dose, some drug molecules find their target cells, while other molecules are being distributed, metabolized, and excreted. At the cellular site of action, drugs exert their primary actions. These actions are described in the following section.

The actions of drugs are studied from a number of different perspectives. Each perspective provides

Table 1.3 Renal Processes that Influence Drug Excretion

PROCESS	TRANSPORT ROUTE	DRUGS TRANSPORTED	NOTES
Glomerular Filtration	Drugs pass from the blood into the nephron by perfusing across the fenestrated capillaries of Bowmans Capsule.	Diffusion Process. Small, nonionic drugs pass more readily. Drugs bound to plasma proteins cannot pass.	Rate of filtration depends in part on blood pressure.
Tubular Secretion	Drugs secreted into the nephron tubule from the efferent arteriole.	Active transport (drug carriers and energy). Drugs which specifically bind to carriers (transporters) are transported. Size and charge are less important.	Drugs may compete with one another for the carrier. A drug with a low margin of safety might reach toxic levels. Therapeutically, drugs which compete for transporters can be coadministered to increase plasma half-life.
Tubular Reabsorption	Drugs are reabsorbed into the blood stream from the nephron tubule.	Diffusion Process. Small, nonionic drugs pass more readily.	Because ionic agents are poorly reabsorbed, drug metabolites which are more ionic than the parent drug will be passed into the urine more easily. Urinary pH can be purposely altered to increase the rate of drug excretion (e.g., administration of bicarbonate).

different information and uses different terminology. To avoid confusion over terminology, the actions of drugs are presented in three sections: I) pharmacology at the cellular level, II) pharmacology at the organism level, and III) pharmacology at the population level.

• *Pharmacology at the Cellular Level*

Drug Receptors: Receptors are generally proteins or glycoproteins that are present on the cell surface, on an organelle within the cell, or in the cytoplasm. There is a finite number of receptors in a given cell. Thus, receptor-mediated responses plateau upon (or before) receptor saturation. When a drug binds to a receptor, one of the following actions is likely to occur (Fig. 1.3):

• An ion channel is opened or closed.

• Biochemical messengers, often called second messengers, (cAMP, cGMP, Ca^{++}, inositol phosphates) are activated. The biochemical messenger initiates a series of chemical reactions within the cell, which transduce the signal stimulated by the drug.

• A normal cellular function is physically inhibited (e.g., DNA synthesis, bacterial cell wall production, protein synthesis).

• A cellular function is "turned on" (e.g., steroid promotion of DNA transcription).

Very precise terminology is required when discussing drug-receptor interactions. It is also important to avoid substituting terms that describe drug actions at the organism or population level (e.g., potency, efficacy, therapeutic index) for terms describing drug actions at the receptor level (e.g., affinity).

The Receptor Theory of Drug Action: Langley and Ehrlich first proposed that drug actions were mediated by chemical receptors. In 1933, Clark developed the dose-response theory which stated that increased response to a drug depended on increased binding of drug to receptors. In 1956, Stephenson presented a modified dose-response theory which is more widely accepted today.

• Clark's Theory

1. Drug response is proportional to the number of receptors occupied.

2. Assumed that all drug-receptor interactions were reversible.

3. Assumed that drug binding to receptors represented only a fraction of available drug.

4. Assumed that each receptor bound only one drug.

- **Stephenson's modified theory** (generally accepted)
  1. Drug response depends on both the affinity of a drug for its receptors (defined below) and the drug's efficacy (defined in the next section).
  2. Described **spare receptors.** Proposed that maximal response can be achieved even if a fraction of receptors (spare receptors) are unoccupied.

The following terminology refers only to events which occur at the cellular level:

- **Affinity:** Affinity refers to the STRENGTH of binding between a drug and its receptor. The number of cell receptors occupied by a drug is a function of an equilibrium between drug which is bound to receptors and drug that is free. A high-affinity agonist or antagonist is less likely than a low-affinity drug to dissociate from a receptor once it is bound.

- **Dissociation Constant (K_D):** The dissociation constant is the measure of a drug's affinity for a given receptor. It is the concentration of drug required in solution to achieve 50% occupancy of its receptors. Units are expressed in molar concentration.

- **Agonist:** Drugs which alter the physiology of a cell by binding to plasma membrane or intracellular receptors. Usually, a number of receptors must be occupied by agonists before a measurable change in

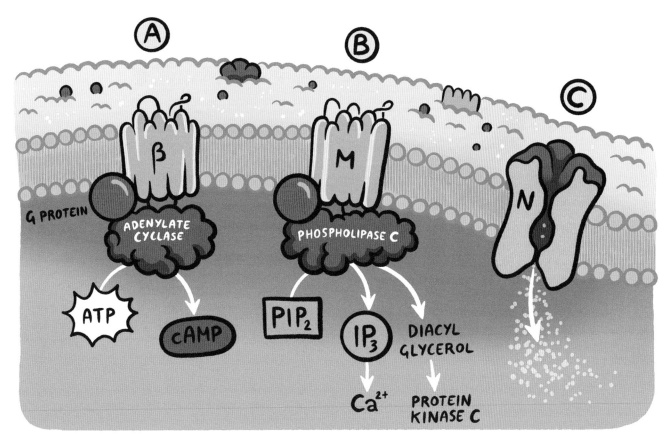

Figure 1.3 Examples of receptors and associated biochemical (second) messenger systems or ion channels. ***A).*** *Receptors such as the beta-adrenergic receptor (β) are coupled with adenylate cyclase through a "G protein" (so named because it binds GTP). When an agonist binds the receptor, the G protein signals adenylate cyclase to synthesize cyclic adenosine monophosphate (cAMP) which subsequently acts as an intracellular messenger.* ***B).*** *Receptors such as the muscarinic acetylcholine receptor (M) are coupled with a G protein that stimulates phospholipase C. Phospholipase C catalyzes the breakdown of phosphatidyl inositol 5,5-bisphosphate (PIP_2) to produce inositol trisphosphate (IP_3) and diacylglycerol (DAG). IP_3 may in turn stimulate other intracellular messengers, such as calcium or calmodulin and DAG stimulates protein kinase C. Protein kinase C acts by phosphorylating target proteins.* ***C).*** *Some receptors regulate ion channels in the plasma membrane. When the nicotinic receptor (N) is stimulated by acetylcholine, the channel opens and sodium ions pass into the cell. In the example of the nicotinic receptor, the drug receptor is a component of the proteins that form the ion channel. In other cases, a distinct receptor might be linked to the ion channel by a G protein or other biochemical messengers.*

cell function occurs. For example, a muscle cell does not depolarize simply because one molecule of acetylcholine binds to a nicotinic receptor and activates an ion channel.

- **Strong Agonist:** An agonist which causes maximal effects even though it may only occupy a small fraction of receptors on a cell.
- **Weak Agonist:** An agonist which must be bound to many more receptors than a strong agonist to produce the same effect.
- **Partial Agonist:** A drug which fails to produce maximal effects, even when all the receptors are occupied by the partial agonist.
- **Antagonist:** Antagonists inhibit or block responses caused by agonists.
- **Competitive Antagonist:** Competes with agonists for receptors. During the time that a receptor is occupied by an antagonist, agonists cannot bind to the receptor. The number of receptors appears unchanged because high doses of agonists will compete for essentially all the receptors. The agonists affinity, however, appears lower because a higher dose of agonist is required, in the presence of antagonist, to achieve receptor occupancy. Because the antagonism can be overcome by high doses of agonists, competitive antagonism is said to be **surmountable.**
- **Noncompetitive Antagonist:** Binds to a site other than the agonist-binding domain. Induces a conformational change in the receptor such that the agonist no longer "recognizes" the agonist-binding domain. Even high doses of agonist cannot overcome this antagonism. Thus it is considered to be **insurmountable.** The number of agonist-binding sites *appears* to be reduced, but the affinity of agonist for the "unantagonized sites" remains unchanged.
- **Irreversible Antagonist (Nonequilibrium competitive):** Irreversible antagonists are also **insurmountable.** These agents compete with agonists for the agonist-binding domain. In contrast to competitive antagonists, however, irreversible antagonists combine permanently with the receptor. The rate of antagonism can be slowed by high concentrations of agonist. Once an irreversible antagonist binds to a particular receptor, however, that receptor cannot be "reclaimed" by an agonist.

   Other forms of antagonism: In addition to pharmacologic antagonism, there are two other mechanisms by which a drug can inhibit or block the effects of an agonist:

- **Physiological Antagonism:** Two agonists, in unrelated reactions, cause opposite effects. The effects cancel one another.

- **Antagonism by Neutralization:** Two drugs bind to one another. When combined, both drugs are inactive.

   Chemicals that are produced in the body and exert their actions through receptors (e.g., acetylcholine, insulin) are termed endogenous ligands.

• *Pharmacology at the Organism Level*

   Many of the terms used in pharmacology were developed to reflect the observations made following administration of a drug to an experimental animal or to a person. The following terms describe the actions of drugs on whole organisms. These terms are more likely to be used in a clinical setting than terms relating to drug-receptor interactions.

   Efficacy: The degree to which a drug is able to induce maximal effects. If Drug A reduces blood pressure by 20 mm and Drug B reduces blood pressure by 10 mm, then Drug A has greater efficacy than Drug B. In this case, Drug A might be appropriate for treating hypertension that is refractory to Drug B.

   Potency: The amount of drug required to produce 50% of the maximal response that the drug is capable of inducing. For example, morphine and codeine are both capable of relieving post-operative pain. A smaller dose of morphine than codeine is required to achieve this effect. Therefore, morphine is more potent than codeine.

   "Potency" and "efficacy" have different meanings and are used to describe different phenomenon. The term "potency" is frequently used to compare drugs within a chemical class, such as narcotic analgesics or corticosteroids. These drugs usually have similar maximal efficacy, if a high enough dose is given.

   "Efficacy" is more easily used to compare drugs with different mechanisms. For example, ketorolac (a nonsteroidal antiinflammatory drug) has equal efficacy to morphine in controlling post-operative pain. Acetaminophen or aspirin have a lower efficacy than either of the above drugs for controlling post-operative pain.

   Nothing can be said about the affinity of drugs based on their efficacy or potency. Affinity is a measure of the "strength" of binding between the drug and its receptor and cannot be measured clinically. A low affinity agonist might produce a response equal to or greater than that produced by a high affinity agonist. Antagonists do not have efficacy, since they do not produce responses.

   Graded dose-response curves: Graphs the magnitude of drug actions against the concentration (or dose) of drug required to induce those actions. The curve represents the effects and dose of a drug within an individual animal or tissue rather than in a population. The receptor affinity, absorption, plasma protein binding, distribution, metabolism, and excretion of a drug all affect the dose response curve.

• Pharmacology at the Population Level

Before new drugs can be approved for marketing, their efficacy and safety must be tested in animal and human population studies. Data derived from these studies are presented using the following terminology:

- **EC_{50} (Effective Concentration 50%):** The concentration of drug which induces a specified clinical effect in 50% of the subjects to which the drug is administered.
- **LD_{50} (Lethal Dose 50%):** The concentration of drug which induces death in 50% of the subjects to which the drug is administered.
- **Therapeutic Index:** A measure of the safety of a drug. Calculated by dividing the LD_{50} by the ED_{50}.
- **Margin of Safety:** The margin between therapeutic and lethal doses of a drug.

Drug Interactions

Drugs may interact with one another according to the following mechanisms:

- **Altered absorption:** Drugs may inhibit absorption of other drugs across biologic membranes (e.g., antiulcer agents that coat the stomach may decrease GI absorption of other drugs).
- **Altered metabolism:** Clinically important drug interactions can occur when the P450 isoenzymes (chemical cousins) are inhibited or induced. CYP is the cytochrome nomenclature used to describe the human P450 isoenzyme followed by the family (an Arabic number), followed by subfamily (a capital letter), followed by the individual gene (an Arabic number). Examples include CYP3A4, CYP1A2, and CYP2C9. Drugs and other substrates (such as smoking) can be inducers or inhibitors of the P450 isoenzymes. Other drugs can be substrates for the particular isoenzymes and thus can be candidates for drug interactions. For example, phenobarbital, a potent inducer of isoenzyme CYP3A4 can produce a clinically significant drug interaction with tacrolimus, a CYP3A4 isoenzyme substrate. Higher doses of tacrolimus and more frequent drug monitoring may be required to keep adequate serum concentrations of tacrolimus in the blood stream. An example of inhibition can be described with the two drugs amiodarone and digoxin. Amiodarone is a potent inhibitor of isoenzymes CYP2C9 and CYP2D6. Because digoxin is a substrate for one of these isoenzymes, amiodarone may produce an increase in the digoxin serum level more than two-fold.

- **Plasma protein competition (Fig. 1.1):** Drugs that bind to plasma proteins may compete with other drugs for the protein binding sites. Displacement of a 'Drug A' from plasma proteins by 'Drug B' may increase the concentration of unbound 'Drug A' to toxic levels.
- **Altered excretion:** Drugs may act on the kidney to reduce excretion of specific agents (e.g., probenecid competes with sulfonamides for the same carrier, increasing the risk of sulfonamide toxicity).

Addition, synergism, potentiation or antagonism are the terms used to describe drug interactions. Table 1.4 demonstrates the differences between the four types of drug interactions.

Tolerance, Dependence and Withdrawal

Tolerance represents a decreased response to a drug. Clinically, it is seen when the dose of a drug must be increased to achieve the same effect. Tolerance can be

Table 1.4 Types of Drug Interactions

TYPE OF INTERACTION	MATHEMATICAL MODEL
Addition – The response elicited by combined drugs is EQUAL TO the combined responses of the individual drugs.	1 + 1 = 2
Synergism – The response elicited by combined drugs is GREATER THAN the combined responses of the individual drugs.	1 + 1 = 3
Potentiation – A drug which has no effect enhances the effect of a second drug.	0 + 1 = 2
Antagonism – Drug inhibits the effect of another drug. Usually, the antagonist has no inherent activity.	1 + 1 = 0

metabolic (drug is metabolized more rapidly after chronic use), *cellular* (decreased number of drug receptors, known as **downregulation**), or *behavioral* (an alcoholic learns to hide the signs of drinking to avoid being caught by his colleagues).

Dependence occurs when a patient needs a drug to "function normally". Clinically, it is detected when cessation of a drug produces withdrawal symptoms. Dependence can be physical (chronic use of laxatives leads to dependence on laxatives to have a normal bowel movement) or may have a psychological component (Do you HAVE to drink a cup of coffee to start your day?).

Withdrawal occurs when a drug is no longer administered to a dependent patient. The symptoms of withdrawal are often the opposite of the effects achieved by the drug (cessation of antihypertensive agents frequently causes severe hypertension and reflex tachycardia). In some cases, such as withdrawal from morphine or alcohol, symptoms are complex and may seem unrelated to drug effects.

Cross tolerance/cross dependence occurs when tolerance or dependence develops to different drugs which are chemically or mechanistically related. For example, methadone relieves the symptoms of heroin withdrawal because patients develop cross dependence to these two drugs.

The Patient Profile

The Importance of the patient profile: Prescribing drugs without consideration for the patient profile is substandard care. The patient profile includes each of the following considerations:

- **Age:** Drug metabolizing enzymes are often undeveloped in infants and depressed in the elderly. Because drugs are not metabolized as readily, they may accumulate to toxic concentrations. Pediatric and geriatric dosing regimens are provided by most drug manufacturers. It is *inappropriate* to extrapolate adult doses to children. Instead, pediatric dosing regimens are available for most drugs and are usually adjusted according to patient weight or body surface area.

- **Pregnancy status:** Before prescribing drugs for a woman of child-bearing age, it is essential to know *whether there is any possibility* that she is pregnant or whether she is nursing. Many drugs are not to be prescribed for pregnant or nursing women. Others may be administered with caution.

- **Smoking and drinking habits:** Both smoking and drinking induce P450 liver enzymes. This accelerates the metabolism of a number of drugs. In some cases, the result is lower-than-expected drug concentration, leading to decreased therapeutic effectiveness. Prodrugs, however, might be metabolized to more active forms. In some cases, the active drug reaches toxic concentrations.

- **Liver or kidney disease:** Dose reduction may be necessary in patients with liver or kidney dysfunction. Failing kidneys excrete fewer drug metabolites. Failing livers metabolize drugs poorly compared to properly functioning livers. Liver and kidney failure are particularly common in the geriatric population.

- **Pharmacogenetics:** This is the most difficult assessment in the patient profile. Briefly, there are genetic differences between patients which affect the pharmacokinetics and actions of many drugs. For example, the half-life of phenytoin ranges from 10 hours in a "high hydroxylator" to 42 hours in a "low hydroxylator" simply because the level of microsomal hydroxylation is lower in the latter patient. A number of specific pharmacogenetic traits have been described. Specific traits, associated mechanisms, and pharmacogenetic methodology are not discussed in this introductory chapter.

- **Drug interactions**

- **Psychosocial factors:** Poor patient compliance is the cause of many 'drug failures'. Before prescribing a medication, consider the cost, ease of administration, and dose schedule of the drug. Also, assess the level of patient responsibility.

Chapter 2 **Peripheral Nervous System**

The **peripheral nervous system** is divided into the autonomic and somatic nervous systems. The **autonomic nervous system** controls cardiac and smooth muscle contraction, and glandular secretion. The **somatic nervous system** supplies skeletal muscle during voluntary movement and conducts sensory information, such as pain and touch.

The autonomic nervous system is further divided into the sympathetic and parasympathetic systems, which generally oppose one another. For example, the **sympathetic system** is generally catabolic, expending energy (the "fight or flight system"). It increases heart rate, dilates bronchi, and decreases secretions, whereas the **parasympathetic system** is anabolic, conserving energy. e.g., it decreases heart rate, stimulates gastrointestinal function (See Figs. 2.2 and 2.3 for a review of functions). In the resting individual, the parasympathetic system dominates in most organs, resulting in a relatively slow heartbeat, adequate secretions, and appropriate bowel motility. In an individual under stress, however, the sympathetic system dominates, diverting energy to functions which make a person fit to fight or flee (e.g., improved oxygenation of tissues by bronchodilation and increased cardiac output).

Autonomic neurotransmission involves two neurons, the preganglionic and the postganglionic neurons (Fig. 2.1). Preganglionic neurons extend from the brain to autonomic ganglia where they transmit CNS signals to postganglionic neurons by releasing acetylcholine into the synaptic cleft, which is the space between the two neurons. Postganglionic neurons subsequently transmit impulses to end organs (e.g., heart, stomach) by releasing norepinephrine (sympathetic neurons) or acetylcholine (parasympathetic neurons).

The **catecholamines** norepinephrine and epinephrine transmit most impulses of the sympathetic system. Upon release from postganglionic neurons, **norepinephrine** diffuses across the synaptic cleft and binds to postsynaptic adrenergic ($\alpha 1$, $\alpha 2$, $\beta 1$ or $\beta 2$) receptors. During times of stress, the adrenal gland releases **epinephrine** (adrenaline) into the blood. Like norepinephrine, circulating epinephrine is an agonist at adrenergic (sympathetic) receptors. An exception to catecholamine neurotransmission in the sympathetic system is the sweat glands. Acetylcholine, which is often considered a parasympathetic transmitter, conveys sympathetic signals to sweat glands.

Acetylcholine transmits all parasympathetic signals to end organs (heart, lungs, etc.) by binding to **muscarinic (M) receptors**. In addition, acetylcholine plays three other important roles in neurotransmission.

- **Ganglionic transmission:** Acetylcholine transmits both sympathetic and parasympathetic impulses from the preganglionic neurons in the brain and spinal cord to **nicotinic ganglionic (N_g) receptors** on postganglionic neurons of the autonomic nervous system. This occurs in sympathetic ganglia, which are located along the spinal cord, and in parasympathetic ganglia, which lie near the end organs. Because all

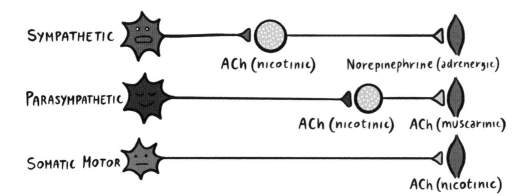

SYMPATHETIC — ACh (nicotinic) — Norepinephrine (adrenergic)

PARASYMPATHETIC — ACh (nicotinic) — ACh (muscarinic)

SOMATIC MOTOR — ACh (nicotinic)

Figure 2.1 Schematic of autonomic and somatic motor neurons. Presynaptic neurons are depicted with solid cell bodies. Postsynpatic neurons are speckled. The neurotransmitter released by the presynaptic neuron and the type of receptor it activates are listed below each synapse.

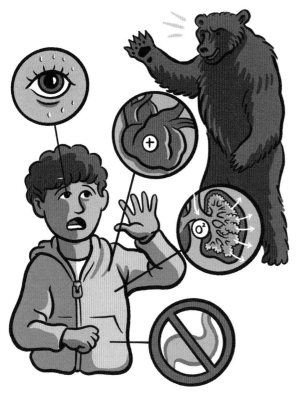

Figure 2.2 The "Fight or Flight" response demonstrates the ability of the sympathetic nervous system to provide energy for vital functions. Decreased pulmonary secretions and bronchodilation increase blood oxygenation. Increased heart rate and contractility improve cardiac output. Arteriolar constriction shunts blood from the skin and digestive tract, whereas arterioles in the heart and skeletal muscle dilate to supply more blood to the latter organs. Glycogen and lipids break down and glucose is synthesized for energy. GI motility and secretions decrease and urine is retained (because you can't fight a bear when you're urinating).

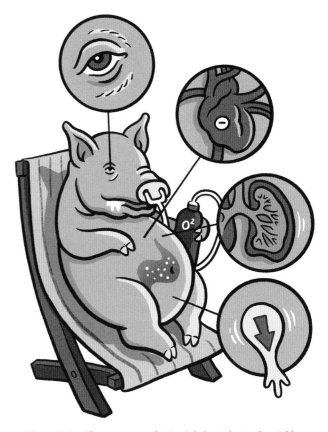

Figure 2.3 The parasympathetic pig's heart beats sluggishly while his digestive tract hogs the energy. He's drooling because of increased secretions. He needs to breath oxygen because his bronchioles are constricted. He is defecating and urinating and he has an erection (you'll have to picture this as none of these are drawn, for modesty). (The sympathetic system, by the way, controls ejaculation). Notice how tiny his pupils are compared to the scared boy in figure 2.2.

ganglionic transmission is cholinergic, drugs which block ganglionic transmission (Table 2.8) inhibit either sympathetic or parasympathetic signals, depending on which system is predominant at the moment.

- **Neuromuscular transmission**: Acetylcholine, released from neurons, causes muscle contraction by binding to **nicotinic muscle (N_m)** receptors on muscle cells, causing calcium influx (Fig. 2.1).

- **Central neurotransmission:** Acetylcholine is a neurotransmitter in the brain, acting predominantly via muscarinic receptors.

Before learning about specific drugs which modify neurotransmission, it is helpful to consider how messages are transmitted from one neuron to another and the strategies available for enhancing or suppressing neurotransmission.

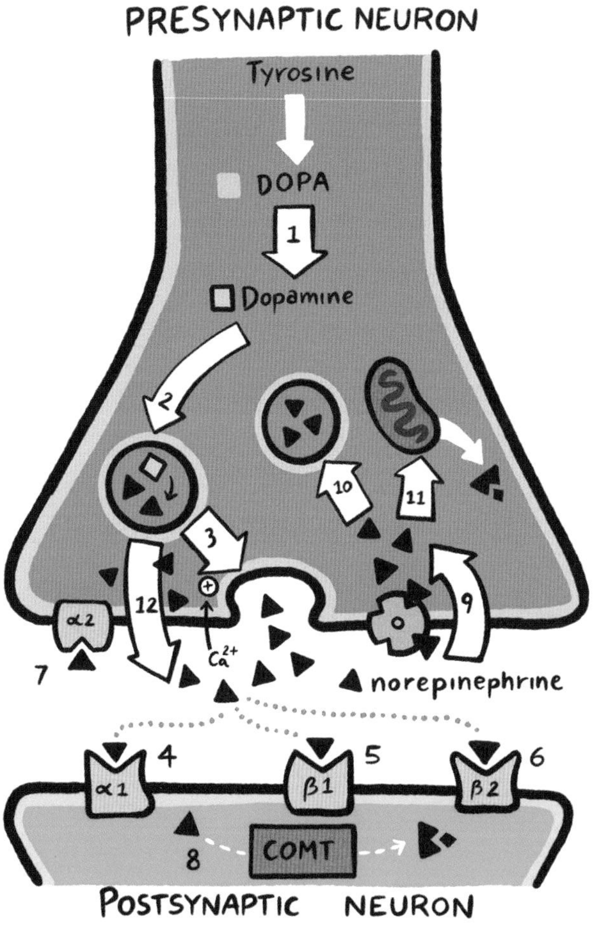

PRESYNAPTIC NEURON

Tyrosine

DOPA

1

Dopamine

2

10 11

3

12

α2

7   Ca²⁺   ▲ norepinephrine

9

o

4   5   6
α1   β1   β2

8   COMT

POSTSYNAPTIC   NEURON

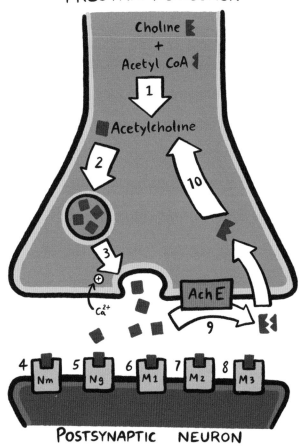

PRESYNAPTIC NEURON

Choline
+
Acetyl CoA

1

Acetylcholine

2

10

3

Ca²⁺   AchE

9

4   5   6   7   8
Nm   Ng   M1   M2   M3

POSTSYNAPTIC   NEURON

Figure 2.4A Norepinephrine synthesis, release and degradation.
1). Norephinephrine is synthesized from the amino acid tyrosine. Tyrosine is hydroxylated to dopa which is then decarboxylated to dopamine. 2). Dopamine (empty squares) diffuses into synaptic vesicles where the enzyme dopamine β-hydroxylase hydroxylates dopamine, forming norepinephrine (solid squares). 3). Upon nerve stimulation, calcium enters the presynaptic neuron and causes the synaptic vesicles to fuse with the plasma membrane and release norepinephrine into the synaptic cleft. 4, 5, 6). Norepinephrine diffuses throughout the synaptic space and may bind to either α1 adrenergic receptors, β1 adrenergic receptors or β2 adrenergic receptors. Direct sympathomimetic drugs (adrenergic agonists) bind to these receptors as well, without interacting with the presynaptic neuron. 7). α2 adrenergic receptors are located on the presynaptic neuron in some cases. Stimulation of α2 presynaptic receptors by norepinephrine inhibits subsequent release of norepinephrine from the terminal. 8). The enzyme catechol-o-methyl transferase degrades catecholamines, such as norepinephrine. 9). More commonly, excess norepinephrine is transported back into the presynaptic neuron where it is (10) repackaged in storage vesicles or (11) degraded by mitochondrial monoamine oxidase. 12). Indirect sympathomimetics are drugs that work by entering the presynaptic terminal and displacing norepinephrine.

First, consider the processes involved in neurotransmission (Fig. 2.4A and 2.4B): 1) the neurotransmitter is synthesized from chemical precursors, 2) it is packaged into vesicles in the presynaptic terminal, 3) the presynaptic nerve is stimulated causing the synaptic vesicles to fuse with the synaptic membrane and release the

Figure 2.4B Synthesis, release and degradation of acetylcholine.
1). The enzyme choline acetyltransferase catalyzes the acetylation of choline by acetyl CoA to form acetylcholine. 2). Acetylcholine is stored in storage vesicles. 3). Upon nerve stimulation, an action potential travels down the neuron and causes calcium influx into the nerve terminal. Calcium influx causes the vesicles to fuse with plasma membrane and release acetylcholine. Acetylcholine diffuses through the synaptic cleft and may bind to (4) Nm receptors (nicotinic receptors on muscle cells, (5) Ng receptors (nicotinic receptors on ganglionic synapses of the autonomic nervous system), (6) M1 muscarinic receptors, (7) M2 muscarinic receptors or (8) M3 muscarinic receptors. At least six muscarinic receptors have now been identified, of which M1, M2 and M3 receptors have been most carefully studied (Table 2.5). 9). Acetylcholine is cleared from the synaptic cleft by acetylcholinesterase (AChE) hydrolysis to choline, which is actively reabsorbed into the nerve terminal. 10). Acetylcholine breakdown products are recycled into acetylcholine.

neurotransmitter, 4) the neurotransmitter diffuses across the synaptic cleft and may bind to postsynaptic receptors, 5) binding of neurotransmitter to receptor results in either opening of an ion channel or activation of a "second messenger" such as cAMP or inositol phosphate, 6) the resulting ion influx or second messenger activation causes an action (e.g., depolarization) of the postsynaptic cell. Neurotransmitter molecules which fail to bind to postsynaptic receptors are destroyed by degradative enzymes, are taken up into the presynaptic neuron to be recycled, or diffuse away from the synaptic cleft.

Clinically useful agents which enhance neurotransmission include:

- **Receptor agonists**
- **Agents which induce neurotransmitter release**
- **Drugs which prevent transmitter degradation**

Clinically useful agents which suppress neurotransmission include:

- **Presynaptic nerve blockers**
- **Receptor antagonists**
- **Ganglion blockers**

Sympathomimetics
• Direct Sympathomimetics

Endogenous sympathetic agonists (norepinephrine, epinephrine and dopamine) and other sympathomimetic drugs are presented in Tables 2.1A and 2.1B. Direct sympathetic agonists bind to α_1, α_2, β_1, or β_2 adrenergic receptors where they "turn on" second messengers (Fig. 2.5). The second messenger associated with each receptor class mediates different effects. Thus the actions of each agonist depend on the class or classes of receptors to which it binds and the tissue location of the receptors.

Table 2.1A Direct Sympathomimetics

DRUG	RECEPTOR	VASCULAR EFFECTS	CARDIAC EFFECTS
Catecholamines:			
Epinephrine (Adrenalin)	α and β	Vasoconstriction (α1). Vasodilation (β2). Injected with local anesthetics: α1-mediated vasoconstriction delays distribution of anesthetic away from the site of injection.	All cardiac effects mediated by β1 receptors: Increased heart rate; contractility; conduction velocity; and automaticity of A-V node, HIS-Purkinje fibers and ventricles.
Norepinephrine (Levophed)	$\alpha > \beta1 >> \beta2$	α1: INTENSE vasoconstriction leading to ↑↑ mean arterial pressure. (vasoconstriction is unopposed because drug fails to bind to β2 receptors – which cause vasodilation when stimulated).	Intense vasoconstriction causes reflex (parasympathetic-mediated) slowing of the heart. This reflex bradycardia overwhelms the weak β1 cardiostimulatory effects.
Isoproterenol (Isuprel)	Only β	Intense vasodilation (β2) reduces mean arterial pressure. Doesn't bind to α1 receptors.	Stimulates heart more than epinephrine due to direct effects and response to decreased mean arterial pressure.
Dobutamine (Dobutrex)	$\beta1 > \beta2 = \alpha$	NO CHANGE in resistance because it has low affinity for α1 and β2.	Drug of choice to stimulate heart. Preserves the heart's efficiency best. Minor change in heart rate.
Dopamine (Intropin)	Dopamine receptors and β1 adrenergic receptors	Low doses: constricts arterioles in sites other than the brain & kidneys. Thus preserves flow to these vital organs. At higher doses, constricts all vessels.	β1 effects: ↑ contractility, ↑ systolic pressure, less effect on rate than isoproterenol. Causes indirect release of norepinephrine which is offset by inhibition of norepinephrine release via presynaptic dopamine receptors.
Noncatecholamines:			
Phenylephrine (Neo-Synephrine)	Primarily α	Intense vasoconstriction. ↑ mean arterial pressure.	↓ heart rate (reflex to ↑ mean arterial pressure). Used clinically to treat paroxysmal supraventricular tachycardia.
Methoxamine (Vasoxyl)	" "	" "	" "
Metaproterenol (Alupent)	Primarily β2.	Vasodilation.	Very few cardiac effects due to lack of affinity for β1 receptors.
Albuterol (e.g., Ventolin) **Bitolterol** (Tornalate) **Terbutaline** (Brethine) **Salmeterol** (Serevent) **Pirbuterol** (Maxair) **Levalbuterol** (Xopenex)	" " " " " " " " " " " "	" " " " " " " " " " " "	" " " " " " " " " " " "
See Table 5.1A for additional bronchodilators			

The location of adrenergic receptors and the consequences of their stimulation are outlined in Table 2.2.

Catecholamines are chemicals which contain a catechol group and an amine. Catechol-O-methyl transferase (COMT) and monoamine oxidase (MAO) are degradative enzymes which rapidly metabolize catecholamines and consequently shorten the duration of catecholamine effects. Despite their short duration of action, catecholamines are used clinically to treat anaphylaxis, cardiac arrest, heart failure and shock (Table 4.2B and associated text).

Noncatecholamine adrenergic agonists (Table 2.1A) have longer serum half-lives than catecholamines, because they are not metabolized by MAO or COMT. Most noncatecholamine sympathomimetics are β_2-preferring agents which are marketed as bronchodilators (Table 2.1A) or uterine relaxants (Table 10.3).

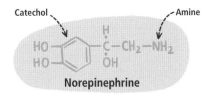

PULMONARY	METABOLIC	OTHER EFFECTS	NOTES
Bronchodilation (β), vasoconstriction (α), and decreased secretions (α). Used therapeutically as bronchodilator (Table 5.1).	Glycogenolysis and gluconeogenesis (β2), lipolysis (β1), predominant ↓ insulin release (α2) but also ↑ insulin release (β2), ↑ renin secretion (β1)	Gut relaxation (α, β2); bladder sphincter contraction (α); uterus contraction in non-pregnant women (α1), uterus relaxation in near-term women (β2).	
No β2 effects. Thus it cannot be used as a bronchodilator.	Relatively weak ↓ insulin release (α2), lipolysis (β1).		Endogenous transmitter of the peripheral nervous system. Used only when intense vasoconstriction is necessary (septic shock).
Clinically used to prevent bronchospasm. Most potent bronchodilator	↑ glycogenolysis and gluconeogenesis, hyperglycemia, hyperlipidemia. ↑ insulin release.	↓ tone and motility of gut. Inhibits mast cell release.	Metabolized by COMT, but it is a poor substrate for monoamine oxidase.
			Synthetic derivative of dopamine, but has no effect at dopamine receptors.
		In kidney, ↑ glomerular filtration rate, ↑ blood flow, ↑ Na⁺ excretion.	Clinically used to treat shock (underperfusion, reflex vasoconstriction).
		Included in cold remedies as a nasal decongestant. Decongestant effects due to nasal vasoconstriction.	Used to treat paroxysmal atrial tachycardia. Reflex ↓ heart rate is maintained after drug is removed.
			" "
Clinically used as a bronchodilator (Table 5.1).		CNS-tremor	Relax uterus in near term pregnant women.
" "			
" "		CNS-tremor	
" "			
" "			
" "			
" "			Long-acting (Salmeterol)

17

Exceptions include phenylephrine and methoxamine which are potent α_1 vasopressors. Phenylephrine is marketed as nasal and ophthalmic decongestants.

• *Indirect & Mixed Agents*

Indirect sympathomimetics cause norepinephrine release from presynaptic terminals, but do not bind to adrenergic receptors (Fig. 2.5, Table 2.1B). These drugs enter the presynaptic terminal and displace stores of norepinephrine from storage vesicles. Mixed sympathomimetics displace norepinephrine from presynaptic terminals *and* bind to adrenergic receptors. (Fig. 2.5, Table 2.1B).

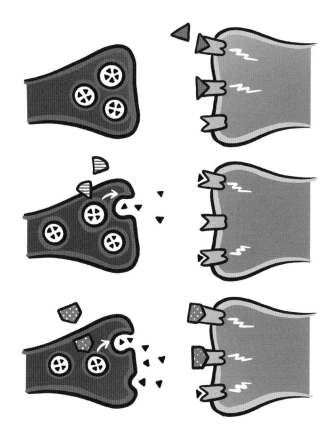

Figure 2.5 Direct, indirect and mixed actions of sympathomimetic drugs. *TOP: Direct agents (open triangles) mimic norepinephrine as agonists at adrenergic receptors without interacting with the presynaptic neuron. The chemical structure of the drug determines its subclass specificity. MIDDLE: Indirect sympathomimetics (striped) force epinephrine release from the presynaptic terminal (solid triangles). Thus, these agents* enhance *the actions of endogenous norepinephrine. Indirect agents do not bind to adrenergic receptors. BOTTOM: Mixed sympathomimetics (speckled) induce the release of norepinephrine and also bind to adrenergic receptors. Sympathetic neurotransmission is also enhanced by inhibition of the degradative enzyme, monoamine oxidase. Monoamine oxidase inhibitors are used to treat depression (Table 3.1B).*

Table 2.1B Indirect and Mixed Sympathomimetics

DRUG	VASCULAR EFFECTS	CARDIAC EFFECTS	CNS EFFECTS
Indirect Agents:			
Amphetamine	Vasoconstriction (due to release of norepinephrine) ↑ mean arterial pressure.	↑ contraction (β1). ↓ heart rate (reflex to ↑ mean arterial pressure)	Wakefulness, elation, ↓ appetite, improved simple motor tasks, euphoria.
Methamphetamine	" "	" "	" "
Mixed agents:			
Ephedrine	Vasoconstriction (α1)– ↑ mean arterial pressure.	Similar to epinephrine, but no change in heart rate.	Clinically used to treat narcolepsy.
Hydroxy-amphetamine	" "	" "	More CNS effects than ephedrine, fewer CNS effects than amphetamine.

Table 2.2 Location and Effects of Stimulation of Adrenergic Receptors

ALPHA -1 RECEPTORS	ALPHA -2 RECEPTORS
Smooth muscle: contraction	**Presynaptic:** ↓ norepinephrine release
Arterioles and veins: Vasoconstriction	CNS: ↓ sympathetic outflow
Radial muscle of eye: Contraction (Pupil dilation)	
Bladder sphincter: Contraction (Urine retention)	**Postsynaptic:** Inhibitory
Pregnant Uterus: Contraction	CNS: ↓ sympathetic outflow
Glands: ↑ secretion	**Pancreatic islet β cells:** ↓ insulin secretion
Intestines: ↓ motility	
Penis: Ejaculation	

BETA -1 RECEPTORS	BETA -2 RECEPTORS
Heart:	**Smooth muscle:** relaxation
↑ heart rate (SA node)	Trachea and bronchioles: bronchodilation
↑ contractility	Uterus: relaxation
↑ conduction velocity	Arterioles (except skin and brain): dilation
↑ automaticity	Veins: dilation
	Ciliary muscle of the eye: relaxation (minor effect on pupil dilation)
Kidney:	Urinary bladder: detrusor relaxation (minor effect on urine retention)
↑ renin secretion	
	Skeletal muscle: ↑ size, tremor

OTHER EFFECTS	CLINICAL USES	UNDESIRABLE EFFECTS	NOTES
Stunts growth.	Narcolepsy, hyperkinetic syndrome of children, attention deficit disorder, Parkinson's disease.	Hypertension, cerebral hemorrhage, convulsions, coma, confusion, anxiety, hallucinations, fever, tremor, restlessness.	Treat toxicity by acidification of urine (it is a weak base) and administration of α blockers or nitroprusside (for hypertension), and antianxiety agents.
" "	" "	" "	" "
Bronchodilation (direct effect, remember that norepinephrine doesn't cause bronchodilation).	Asthma, nasal congestion, narcolepsy. Used as a mydriatic (dilates pupil).	Less CNS toxicity than amphetamine.	Longer duration, but less potent than epinephrine.
" "			

Sympathetic Blocking Agents (Sympatholytics)

The effects of the sympathetic nervous system can be blocked either by decreasing sympathetic outflow from the brain (Table 2.3), suppressing norepinephrine release from presynaptic neurons (Table 2.3) or blocking postsynaptic adrenergic receptors (Table 2.4).

• Central Sympatholytics

Alpha-2 (α_2) adrenergic receptors *inhibit* sympathetic neurotransmission by two mechanisms. **Postsynaptic α_2 receptors** inhibit sympathetic neurons that exit the brain. Alpha-2 receptors are also found on presynaptic nerve terminals where they inhibit norepinephrine release.

Central sympatholytic drugs are commonly used to treat hypertension (Table 4.3C). Clonidine and guanabenz suppress sympathetic outflow from the brain by binding to α_2 adrenergic receptors. In contrast, methyldopa is metabolized in the presynaptic neuron to α-methyl norepinephrine. When released from the presynaptic terminal, α-methylnorepinephrine acts as a potent α_2 agonist.

Clonidine, guanabenz and methyldopa also prevent norepinephrine release by binding to presynaptic α_2 receptors. The relative contributions of presynaptic and postsynaptic effects of these drugs is not fully known.

• Peripheral Presynaptic Sympatholytics

Peripheral presynaptic sympatholytics inhibit norepinephrine release from the presynaptic terminal. Guanadrel and reserpine deplete norepinephrine from presynaptic vesicles. As a result, guanadrel initially releases norepinephrine from the terminal causing a transient increase in adrenergic transmission.

Table 2.3 Presynaptic Adrenergic Nerve Blockers

DRUG	BLOCKADE MECH	ACTIONS	UNDESIRABLE EFFECTS
Centrally Acting Anti-adrenergics			
Clonidine (Catapres)	Potent α2 AGONIST.	↓ preganglionic sympathetic outflow from brain resulting in ↓ blood pressure.	Orthostatic hypotension. Sedation Rebound hypertension
Guanabenz	" "	" "	" "
Guanfacine (Tenex)	" "	" "	" "
Methyldopa (Aldomet)	Decarboxylated to α-methyl dopamine then β-hydroxy-lated to α-methylnorepinephrine, a potent α2 receptor agonist. Results in ↓ sympathetic outflow from CNS.	↓ preganglionic sympathetic output, rapidly ↓ blood pressure– but sympathetic system can respond with cardiac stimulation.	Sedation, mild orthostatic hypotension, dry mouth, fever, nasal stuffiness, Coombs positive RBCs, salt and water retention, rebound hypertension.
Peripheral Presynaptic Anti-adrenergics			
Guanethidine (Ismelin)	Unknown initial effect. Later, ↓↓ norepinephrine release, ↓ norepinephrine concentration in nerve terminals. Chronically, sensitizes nerve to sympathomimetics.	By rapid IV infusion: ↓ blood pressure, then transient hypertension, then ↓ arterial pressure if patient is standing. ↑ GI motility, fluid retention. Orally: hypotension.	Inhibits ejaculation, diarrhea, orthostatic hypotension. With chronic use, get profound NE depletion and nerve toxicity.
Guanadrel (Hylorel)	" "	" "	" "
Bretylium (Bretylol)	" "	See guanethidine. Prolongs myocardial action potential.	" "
Reserpine	Depletes catecholamines and serotonin in brain, adrenal, and heart. Inhibits uptake of norepinephrine into presynaptic vesicles. Chronically sensitizes patient to sympathomimetics.	Gradual ↓ mean arterial pressure with bradycardia. Antihypertensive effects due to ↓ cardiac output. Tranquilization, sedation.	Nightmares, depression, diarrhea, cramps, ↑ risk of breast cancer, peptic ulcers, parasympathetic predominance.

Reserpine is long-acting, and the postsynaptic neurons respond to the paucity of norepinephrine by "upregulating" (increasing) the number of receptors on the postsynaptic membrane. As a result, the postsynaptic terminal is supersensitive to direct sympathomimetics. Consequently monoamine oxidase inhibitors (which prevent destruction of endogenous catecholamines such as norepinephrine and epinephrine) and direct sympathomimetics (Table 2.1A) should be avoided in patients who have received reserpine.

• Peripheral Postsynaptic Sympatholytics

Alpha-1 blockers: Alpha-1 adrenergic antagonists compete with endogenous catecholamines for binding at α_1 and α_2 receptors. Because norepinephrine and epinephrine cannot bind to a receptor that is occupied by an antagonist, the actions of catecholamines at α adrenergic receptors (Table 2.2) are inhibited. Adrenergic blockers used to treat hypertension are presented in greater detail in Table 4.2C.

The vasodilation induced by alpha-blockers may result in orthostatic hypotension (blood pools in legs when the patient is upright) and tachycardia which is a β_1-mediated sympathetic reflex to hypotension. Because α_2 receptors regulate norepinephrine release, blockade of these receptors might result in hypersecretion of norepinephrine.

Beta blockers: Nonspecific beta blockers (block both β_1 and β_2 receptors) have been used as first-step antihypertensive agents. Because these agents block β_2 receptors as well as β_1 receptors, bronchospasm may occur. Newer agents are β_1-specific and are not contraindicated in asthmatic patients. Some agents have intrinsic sympathomimetic activity (partial agonist activity).

CLINICAL USES	NOTES
Hypertension	
" "	
" "	
Hypertension	
Severe hypertension Renal hypertension	Seldom used
Hypertension	
Arrhythmias	
Hypertension	No rebound effect because effects are long lasting. Sometimes used for noncompliant patients because of long half-life.

Table 2.4 Adrenergic Antagonists

DRUG	RECEPTOR SPECIFICITY	TYPE OF BLOCKADE	ACTIONS
Phenoxy-benzamine (Dibenzyline)	α_1, α_2	Irreversible alkylation of α receptor.	Vasodilation (α_1). Blocks sympathetic outflow from the brain and feedback inhibition of norepinephrine release at α_2 receptors. Increases insulin release
Phentolamine	α_1, α_2	Competitive	Vasodilation
Prazosin (Minipress)	Selective α_1	" "	Vasodilation
Doxazosin (Cardura) **Terazosin**	Selective α_1	" "	Vasodilation
Alfuzosin (Uroxatral) **Tamsulosin** (Flomax)	" "	" "	Vasodilation
Labetalol (Trandate) (Normodyne)	α_1, β_1, β_2	" "	↓ BP (α_1 blockade) without reflex tachycardia (β_1, blockade). Conduction time and refractory period slightly prolonged.
Carvedilol (Coreg)	α_1, β_1, β_2	" "	↓ cardiac output, exercise-induced tachycardia, and reflex orthostatic tachycardia; Vasodilation, ↓ peripheral vascular resistance with ↓ BP
Propranolol (Inderal)	β_1, β_2	" "	Heart: ↓ inotropy, chronotropy, O_2 demand and conduction velocity. Arteries: compensatory vasoconstriction (dwindles over days) Kidney: ↓ β_1 mediated renin release, ↑ Na^+ and H_2O retention Liver: ⇊ glycogenolysis and slows post-insulin recovery of glucose **no change in HR or contractility with pindolol.
Carteolol (Cartrol)	" "	" "	" "
Penbutolol (Levatol)	" "	" "	" "
Sotalol (Betapace)	" "	" "	" "
Nadolol (Corgard)	" "	" "	" "
Timolol (Blocadren)	" "	" "	" "
Pindolol (Visken)	" "	" "	" "
Metoprolol (Lopressor)	β_1 specific	" "	Compared to propranolol; less bronchospasm in asthmatics, less inhibition of vasodilation and liver effects.
Atenolol (Tenormin) **Acebutolol** (Sectral) **Bisoprolol** (Zebeta) **Esmolol** (Brevibloc) **Betaxolol** (Kerlone)	" " " " " " " "	" " " " " " " "	" "

CLINICAL USES	UNDESIRABLE EFFECTS	PHARMACOKINETICS	NOTES
Pheochromocytoma—to control hypertensive episodes.	Postural hypotension (blood pooling), intense reflex tachycardia and force of contraction (enhanced by block of NE feedback control at α_2). Arrhythmias, ischemia, sexual dysfunction, nasal congestion.	Slow onset, but long lasting due to irreversible binding to receptor.	Effects depend on degree of α adrenergic tone.
Pheochromocytoma—to control hypertensive episodes; dermal necrosis; pharmacological test for pheochromocytoma	Tachycardia, cardiac arrhythmias, prolonged hypotensive episodes, nasal congestion, diarrhea.	Rapid onset, short half-life.	
Hypertension.	No large reflex tachycardia; postural hypotension with first dose; less sexual dysfunction.		Tolerance not observed.
Hypertension; benign prostatic hyperplasia (relaxes smooth muscles produced by blockade of α_1 in bladder neck and prostate.	No large reflex tachycardia; postural hypotension with first dose; less sexual dysfunction.	Greater effect on BP and HR in the standing position.	
Benign prostatic hyperplasia.	" "		
Hypertension, IV for severe hypertension.	Further suppresses a failing heart; fatigue, impotence, diarrhea, numbness, orthostatic hypotension.	Oral completely absorbed, with peak levels in 1–2 hr and steady state in 3 days. Extensive 1st pass effect; IV peak occurs in 5 min.	Contraindicated in patients with asthma or bradycardia due to bronchoconstriction.
Essential hypertension, congestive heart failure.	Hepatotoxic, postural hypotension, hypoglycemia.	Well absorbed, extensive 1st pass effect, terminal elimination half-life 7–10 hrs, extensively metabolized.	Contraindicated in patients with asthma due to bronchoconstriction.
Hypertension, angina pectoris, SVT, ventricular arrhythmias, myocardial infarction, migraine prophylaxis, essential tremors and other unlabeled uses.	Further suppresses a failing heart: CNS sedation and depression; rebound hypertension, impotence. Angina, myocardial infarction, arrhythmias may occur if abruptly withdrawn.	Low bioavailability due to significant 1st pass effect; Readily enters CNS; Hall-life 3–5 hours; Hepatically metabolized.	Contraindicated in patients with asthma due to bronchoconstriction. β blockers should be weaned rather than abruptly withdrawn.
Hypertension	Bradycardia, ventricular arrhythmias, dizziness, fatigue, hyperglycemia, hypoglycemia, impotence.	Adjust dose for renal impairment.	Has intrinsic sympathomimetic activity; contraindicated in bronchospasm.
Hypertension	" "		" "
Ventricular arrhythmias and tachycardias.	" "	Not metabolized.	Contraindicated in asthma or bronchospasm, long QT syndrome.
Hypertension; angina pectoris	" "	Fewer CNS effects than propranolol; longer half-life than propranolol.	Contraindicated in asthma or bronchospasm.
Hypertension, myocardial infarction, migraine prophylaxis: Ophthamologic agent used to ↓ intraocular pressure.	" "		" "
Hypertension	" "		Has intrinsic sympathomimetic activity; contraindicated in bronchospasm.
Hypertension, angina pectoris, myocardial infarction.	Lower toxicity than propranolol; less likely to increase peripheral resistance, cause bronchospasm, or inhibit liver metabolism.	Readily enter CNS.	
Hypertension	" "		See Table 4.2C

Cholinomimetics

• Direct Cholinergic Agonists

Acetylcholine is the neurotransmitter of the parasympathetic nervous system, the neuromuscular junction, and autonomic ganglia. In addition, acetylcholine in the brain plays a role in memory formation, motor skills and other important tasks.

Muscarinic receptors (M) mediate end-organ postganglionic parasympathetic and most CNS functions of acetylcholine, whereas nicotinic receptors are found in ganglia (N_g) and at the neuromuscular junction (N_m) and specific CNS regions. Table 2.5 outlines cholinergic actions at muscarinic receptors and nicotinic receptors.

Choline esters are simply choline bound to an acetyl derivative by an ester bond. The ester bond of acetylcholine and related drugs is hydrolyzed by enzymes known as cholinesterases (e.g., acetylcholinesterase). Choline esters are more or less sensitive to cholinesterase deactivation depending on their chemical structure.

Cholinomimetic alkaloids are derived from plants by alkaline extraction. They are chemically distinct

Table 2.5 Cholinergic Agonists (Cholinomimetics)

DRUG	RECEPTOR	ORGAN	ACTION
Acetylcholine (Miochol-E)	Muscarinic type 1 (M_1)	Stomach	↑ acid pepsin in secretion
	M_1	Ganglion	stimulation
	M_1	CNS	neurotransmission
	M_2	SA node	↑ K^+ conduction, slow diastolic depolarization, bradycardia
	M_2	Atria	↓ contractility, ↓ conduction velocity, ↓ refractory period
	M_2	AV node	slows conduction, AV block
	M_2	Lung	bronchoconstriction, ↑ secretion
	M_2	Stomach	↑ motility
	M_2	Bladder	contract detruser, relax sphincter
	M_2	Penis	erection
	M_3	Glands	↑ secretion
	M_3	Eye	miosis, accommodation
	Nicotinic	Skeletal Muscle	contraction
	Nicotinic	Ganglion	stimulation
	Nicotinic	CNS	neurotransmission
Choline Derivatives			
Carbachol (Miostat) (Isopto Carbachol)	" "	" "	" "
Methacholine (Provocholine)	M_1, M_2 and M_3. Weak nicotinic agonist.	See M_1, M_2, and M_3 rows above.	See M_1, M_2, and M_3 rows above.
Bethanechol (Urecholine) (Duvoid)	M_1, M_2 and M_3 and nicotinic agonist.	See M_1, M_2, and M_3 rows above.	See M_1, M_2, and M_3 rows above.
Alkaloids			
Cevimeline	M_1, M_2, M_3.	See M_1, M_2, and M_3 rows above.	See M_1, M_2, and M_3 rows above.
Pilocarpine (Pilocar) (Isopto-Carpine)	M_1, M_2, M_3. Not nicotinic.	See M_1, M_2, and M_3 rows above. Sweat and salivary glands particularly pronounced.	See M_1, M_2, and M_3 rows above.
Nicotine	Nicotinic	See nicotinic rows above	See nicotinic rows above

from the choline esters and are not metabolized by cholinesterases.

Nicotine is the prototypic nicotinic receptor agonist and causes depolarization of the target cell. It is among the most commonly used drugs. Smokers become tolerant to and dependent on its effects. Nicotine stimulates the CNS, releases epinephrine from adrenal glands, and stimulates receptors in ganglia and at the neuromuscular junction. In the latter two cases, persistent nicotine action prevents repolarization and hence leads to functional block. Like ganglion blockers, the action of nicotine at each visceral organ depends on whether the sympathetic or parasympathetic system is predominant at the time.

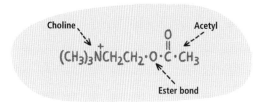

CLINICAL USES	CONTRAINDICATIONS	2ND MESSENGERS	NOTES
Miosis in cataract surgery	Peptic ulcer	At M_1 receptors: G-protein phosphatidyl inositol	
	Coronary artery disease Hyperthyroidism (atrial fibrillation)	At M_2 receptors: ↑ K^+ conduction (SA node), ↓ cAMP (atria and AV node), ↑ cGMP (other organs)	
	Asthma	At M_3 receptors, phosphatidyl inositol	
	Mechanical bladder obstruction	At nicotinic receptor: opens sodium channel. Influx depolarizes cell.	
Glaucoma. Applied topically to the eye.	Where constriction is undesirable	" "	Relatively resistant to cholinesterase degradation (long half-life)
Diagnostic for bronchial airway hyperreactivity without clinically apparent asthma	Patients receiving β-blockers	" "	Short duration of action due to cholinesterase degradation.
To induce evacuation of NON-obstructed bladder. To increase GI motility following surgery.	Above plus bradycardia, parkinsonism, epilepsy, hypotension, hypertension	" "	Relatively specific for gastrointestinal tract and bladder. Resistant to cholinesterase.
Dry mouth associated with Sjogren's Syndrome.	" "	" "	Derived from a seed known as the betel nut
Cystic Fibrosis sweat test, Glaucoma (miotic), Xerostomia	" "	" "	
Smoking cessation aid	" "	" "	The drug initially used to characterize nicotinic pharmacologic responses

Cholinomimetics (cont.)

• Cholinesterase Inhibitors

The actions of acetylcholine are terminated in the synaptic cleft primarily by acetylcholinesterase, which cleaves the transmitter at the ester bond. The agents in Table 2.6 enhance acetylcholine effects at all receptors by inhibiting acetylcholinesterase, thus preventing transmitter (acetylcholine) degradation.

Cholinesterase inhibitors are classified by their mechanism of action.

• The **carbamyl ester inhibitors** compete with acetylcholine for the active site of the enzyme and are poor substrates. Acetylcholinesterase becomes carbamylated as it cleaves the ester linkage. The carbamyl group remains attached for a period of minutes to hours and prevents acetylcholine from binding to the active site of acetylcholinesterase for a period of minutes to hours. Upon decarbamylation, the enzyme regains its ability to cleave acetylcholine.

• The **organophosphorus** inhibitors act in a similar manner and generate an organophosphate modified enzyme that is essentially irreversibly inhibited. Regeneration of the enzyme may take over a week.

Cholinesterase inhibitors are used to treat dementia related to Alzheimer's Disease, glaucoma and myasthenia gravis. Cholinesterase inhibitors do not affect the underlying pathology of Alzheimer's, but increase cholinergic activity in the brain, which may reduce symptoms. In glaucoma, aqueous humor production exceeds outflow, resulting in increased intraocular pressure. In the presence of cholinesterase inhibitor eye drops, acetylcholine causes constriction of the sphincter muscle which surrounds the iris. The iris is drawn away from the canal of Schlemm, enhancing outflow of aqueous humor.

Myasthenia gravis is an autoimmune disease in which antibodies that bind to nicotinic receptors interfere with their number and function at the neuromuscular junction. Cholinesterase inhibitors prevent acetylcholine degrada-

Table 2.6 Cholinesterase Inhibitors

DRUG	MECHANISM	CLINICAL USES	PHARMACOKINETICS
Agents that act in the brain			
Galantamine (Razadyne)	Competitive, reversible cholinesterase inhibitor.	Mild to moderate dementia of Alzheimer's disease.	Crosses the blood brain barrier.
Donepezil (Aricept)	" "	" "	" "
Rivastigmine (Exelon)	" "	" "	" "
Physostigmine	Carbamyl (see text)	Antidote for anticholinergic overdose.	Crosses the blood brain barrier.
Agents that primarily act outside the brain			
Neostigmine (Prostigmine)	Carbamyl	Myasthenia gravis	Ambenonium has more prolonged action than others
Ambenonium (Mytelase)	" "	" "	" "
Pyridostigmine (Mestinon)	" "	" "	" "
Topical agents used for glaucoma			
Demecarium (Humorsol)	Carbamyl	Glaucoma	" "
Echothiophate (Phospholine iodide)	Organophosphorus	Glaucoma	" "

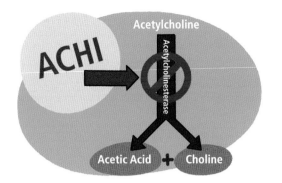

Figure 2.6 Acetylcholinesterase inhibitors (ACHI) prevent acetylcholine degradation by inhibiting the enzyme acetylcholinesterase.

ADMINISTRATION
PO
" "
" "
IM/IV
PO (all) IM/IV (Neostigmine, Pyridostigmine)
" "
" "
Eye drops
Eye drops

tion, which increases the probability that remaining receptors will bind acetylcholine.

Cholinergic Antagonists

Cholinergic **antagonists** are classified as muscarinic blockers (Table 2.7), ganglion blockers, and neuromuscular blockers (Table 2.8). At therapeutic doses, muscarinic antagonists do not bind to nicotinic receptors and neuromuscular blockers (Nm antagonists) do not bind to muscarinic receptors. Most cholinergic **agonists**, on the other hand, bind to both muscarinic and nicotinic receptors.

Muscarinic antagonists, ganglion blockers and neuromuscular blockers are all competitive antagonists which can be overcome by adequate concentrations of cholinergic agonists.

• Muscarinic Antagonists

The prototype antimuscarinic agent is atropine, an alkaloid isolated from *Atropa belladona* (deadly nightshade) and many other plants. Atropine blocks the muscarinic actions of cholinergic agonists (Table 2.5). Its actions are dose dependent, occurring approximately in the following order *as the dose of atropine is increased:*

- Decreased salivary & bronchial secretions
- Decreased sweating (sympathetic controlled)
- Pupil dilation and tachycardia
- Inhibition of voiding (constriction of sphincter and relaxation of detrusor)
- Decreased GI motility
- Decreased gastric secretions

Other muscarinic antagonists resemble atropine, but differ slightly in potency and specificity for various organs. These are noted in table 2.7.

In addition, some antipsychotics, antihistamines, antidepressants, and opioids have anticholinergic effects. Patients receiving these agents should be told that dry mouth, tachycardia and constipation are possible side effects.

Selective muscarinic antagonists used as bronchodilators via inhalation have little systemic effects due to poor absorption and are discussed in Chapter 5.

Belladonna poisoning occurs with the ingestion of anticholinergic drugs or plants such as nightshade, thorn-apple, Jimson weed, stinkweed or devil's apple. Poisoning can also occur in children receiving atropinic eye drops because of systemic absorption.

Symptoms include *severe* antimuscarinic effects (Table 2.7), restlessness, headache, rapid and weak pulse, blurred vision, hallucinations, ataxia, "burning" skin and possibly coma. Children are more susceptible to intoxication and death from belladonna poisoning.

Poisoning is treated with IV physostigmine (Table 2.6). CNS excitement or convulsions may be treated with benzodiazepines.

Cholinergic Antagonists (cont.)

• Ganglion Blockers

Ganglion blockers (Ng antagonists) block nicotinic receptors in both sympathetic and parasympathetic ganglia. Because of the complex and unpredictable

Table 2.7 Muscarinic Antagonists

DRUG	ACTION AT ORGAN	CLINICAL USES
Alkaloids		
Atropine	*Effects at M$_1$ receptors:* • Stomach– ↓ secretion of pepsin and acid *Effects at M$_2$ receptors:* • Heart—low dose—bradycardia (CNS-mediated) • Heart—high dose—tachycardia • CNS– ↓ memory and concentration • Lungs—bronchodilation, ↓ secretion • GI tract– ↓ motility • Eye—cycloplegia, mydriasis, ↑ outflow resistance *Effects at M$_3$ receptors:* • Glands–↓ salivation and sweating	Preanesthetic to prevent respiratory secretions, treatment of parkinsonism, severe bradycardia, peptic ulcers, irritable bowel syndrome, mild diarrhea, bladder spasms, enuresis, bronchospasm
Scopolamine	More potent at eye and glands than atropine, but less potent at heart, lungs and GI tract.	Prevention of motion sickness, nausea and vomiting; inhibits excessive motility of the GI tract in irritable colon syndrome, mild dysentery, diverticulitis.
Synthetic–tertiary compounds:		
Dicyclomine (Bentyl)	Nonspecific direct relaxant effect on smooth muscle; No antimuscarinic activity and thus little effect on gastric acid secretion.	Treatment of irritable bowel syndrome to decrease motility of the bowel.
Oxybutynin (Ditropan)	Direct antispasmodic effect on smooth muscle; no antinicotinic effects. 1/5 of the anticholinergic effect of atropine with 4 to 10 times the antispasmodic activity.	For relief of bladder spasms resulting in urinary leakage and incontinence.
Flavoxate (Urispas)	Relaxes smooth muscle of bladder and also has direct effect on muscle.	Symptomatic relief of dysuria, urgency, nocturia, suprapubic pain, frequency and incontinence that may occur with cystitis, prostatitis, urethritis.
Tolterodine (Detrol)	" "	Treatment of overactive bladder.
Trihexylphenldyl (Artane)	Centrally acting; reduces akinesia, tremor, and rigidity by 20%; may also reduce drooling.	Adjunct treatment of parkinsonism; control of drug-induced extrapyramidal disorders.
Biperiden (Akineton)	" "	" "
Procyclidine (Kemadrin)	" "	" "
Benztropine (Cogentin)	" "	" "
Synthetic–quaternary compounds:		
Methscopolamine bromide (Pamine)	GI	" "
Clidinium bromide	" "	" "
Mepenzolate bromide (Cantil)	" "	" "
Glycopyrrolate (Robinul)	" "	Treatment of peptic ulcer; IV form used to decrease salivary and tracheobronchial secretions and to block cardiac inhibitory reflexes during induction of anesthesia and intubation.

actions of these agents, they are seldom used clinically (Hexamethonium, mecamylamine). Trimethephan is, however, occasionally used to treat hypertensive crisis.

Sympathetic and parasympathetic ganglia are clusters of synapses between the spinal cord and visceral organs in which nerves from the brain connect with nerves which innervate end organs. Acetylcholine is the neurotransmitter in all sympathetic and parasympathetic ganglia. Ganglion blockers therefore reduce the effects of whichever system is predominant. In the resting individual, parasympathetic control dominates all organs except blood vessels and sweat glands.

ADVERSE EFFECTS	PHARMACOKINETICS	NOTES
Dry mouth, urinary retention, tachycardia, CNS-driven bradycardia (general increase in vagal tone). At high doses, CNS excitation (irritability, delerium etc.) followed by CNS depression, possibly resulting in death. Contraindicated in closed angle glaucoma!, open angle glaucoma, prostatic hypertrophy, heart disease, obstructive bowel disease.	Half life 2.5 hrs. Frequent dosing necessary, Eliminated through the urine.	Contraindicated in asthma patients.
More CNS depression than atropine at low doses. Similar to atropine at high doses.	Transdermal preparation has fewer side effects.	Contraindicated if hypersensitive to belladonna or barbiturates.
Tachycardia, headache, flushing, drowsiness, nervousness, dry mouth, constipation, urinary retention.	Little or no antimuscarinic activity with no effect on gastric acid secretion.	Contraindicated in infants < 6 months old.
" " Decreased sweating, rash, decreased lacrimation, mydriasis, cycloplegia.		
" "		
Dry mouth, constipation, headache, dyspepsia, blurred vision.	Reduce dose with liver impairment.	
Tachycardia, hypotension, dry mouth, disorientation, constipation, blurred vision, urinary retention, decreased sweating.	More selective CNS activity than atropine.	
" "	" "	
" "	" "	
" "	" "	
" "	" "	
" "	" "	
" "	" "	
" "	" "	

Thus, when ganglion blockers are administered to nonstressed individuals, one would predict a shift from parasympathetic predominance to sympathetic predominance.

Neuromuscular Blockers

• Neuromuscular Transmission and Blockade

Action potentials trigger calcium influx and the subsequent release of acetylcholine (ACh) from presynaptic motor neurons. ACh diffuses across the membrane cleft and binds to nicotinic receptors on the muscle end plate. Nicotinic receptors have five subunits, two of which bind ACh. When both are occupied, the ion channel (the core of the ring formed by the 5 subunits) opens, allowing Na^+ and Ca^{++} influx and K^+ efflux. The simultaneous opening of many ion channels leads to membrane depolarization and propagation of an action potential in the muscle cell. The action potential induces the excitation-contraction coupling mechanism which causes muscle contraction.

Neuromuscular blockade is classified as nondepolarizing or depolarizing:

• **Nondepolarizing blockade** occurs when pure antagonists compete with agonists for nicotinic receptors.

Because antagonists lack activity, there is no muscle contraction (fasciculations). Blockade is overcome by high concentrations of agonist (ACh).

• **Depolarizing blockade** occurs when an agonist binds to the receptor (causing fasciculations); persistent activation of the receptor prevents repolarization and leads to desensitization, which leads to failed neuromuscular transmission.

Consequence of Blockade: Neuromuscular blockade causes paralysis of all muscles, including those of respiration. Intubation and ventilation equipment must be prepared prior to injecting neuromuscular blockers. Reversing agents must be available.

Monitoring Neuromuscular Blockade: The peripheral nerve stimulator is a device which delivers electrical impulses to nerves by way of electrodes placed on the skin. The response to the stimulus (muscle twitch) indicates the level of neuromuscular blockade.

In the operating room, the most useful stimulation pattern is the **train of four**. Four impulses are delivered over two seconds:

Response:	What response means:
1 twitch	Sufficient relaxation w/nitrous-narcotic
3 twitches	Sufficient relaxation w/inhalation agents
4th twitch > 75% of 1st	Patient ready for extubation

Table 2.8 Neuromuscular Blockers (N_m Antagonists)

DRUG	ACTION	CLINICAL USES	ONSET/DURATION
Competitive Nondepolarizing			
Vecuronium (Norcuron)	Competes with ACh at nicotinic receptors. Does not activate receptor. Blockade can be overcome by high concentration of agonists.	Adjunct to anesthesia: muscle relaxant, eases intubation and ventilation, eases orthopedic manipulation, controls respiration during chest surgery.	Onset: 3–5 min. Duration: 25–40 min.
Atracurium (Tracrium)	" "	Ideal for patients with kidney and liver failure (metabolized in blood).	Onset: 3–5 min. Duration: 20–45 min.
Cisatracurium (Nimbex)	" "	" "	Onset: 2–5 min. Duration: 20–60 min.
Pancuronium (Pavulon)	" " Also has vagolytic actions.	Used when elevated heart rate is desired; Adjunct to anesthesia, to facilitate mechanical ventilation and intubation	Onset: 1–3 min. Duration: 35–55 min.
Rocuronium (Zemuron)	Minimal cardiovascular effect.	Facilitate rapid sequence and routine intubation; Facilitate mechanical ventilation	Onset: 1–3 min. Duration: 15–60 min.
Doxacurium (Nuromax)	" "	Adjunct to anesthesia in long surgery cases; facilitate mechanical ventilation.	Onset: 3–10 min. Duration: 40–240 min.
Competitive Depolarizing			
Succinylcholine (Anectine) (Quelicin)	Initial fasculations (depolarization), then Phase I block (4 min block of voltage sensitive sodium channels). Then, Phase II block (desensitize receptor, lasts 20 min). Parasympathetic stimulation (therapeutic dose), sympathetic stimulation (high dose).	Ideal for intubation because of rapid onset and short duration. Adjunct to anesthesia and mechanical ventilation.	Onset: 30–60 sec, (IV). Duration: 3–5 min.

Other patterns of stimulation include **sustained tetany and single stimulation.** Patients who respond to a sustained (5 second) 50 Hz stimulation are ready for extubation (patient will be able to cough, inspire and raise head). Failure to elicit > 5% of normal twitch to a single 0.2 msec, 0.1 Hz stimulation indicates that the blockade is sufficient for intubation.

• *Reversing Neuromuscular Blockade*

Purpose & timing: Most patients are removed from the ventilator before leaving the surgery suite. Reversal of neuromuscular blockade allows the patient to use the diaphragm and intercostal muscles to breathe. It is essential that at least a single twitch is produced in response to stimulation before an attempt is made to discontinue artificial ventilation.

Pre-reversal: Atropine or glycopyrrolate (muscarinic antagonists (Table 2.7) are often administered prior to reversing agents to prevent bradycardia, salivation and other muscarinic effects caused by the administration of cholinesterase inhibitors.

Reversal: Cholinesterase inhibitors inhibit acetylcholine degradation (Table 2.6). The resulting increased acetylcholine concentration competes with neuromuscular blockers, reversing the blockade. Sugammadex is a reversal agent that binds specifically to rocuronium

and neutralizes its effects. The availability of this reversal agent has made rocuronium the non-depolarizing blocker of choice. Depolarizing neuromuscular agents are used for short term blockade and have a short half-life due to cholinesterase degradation and thus generally do not require a reversal agent.

Local Anesthetics

Local anesthetics are used to block pain conduction by nerves. They are used for infiltration anesthesia, local nerve blocks, spinal nerve blocks and epidural nerve blocks. The first local anesthetic was cocaine, which has largely been replaced by synthetic agents.

Mechanism of Action: Local anesthetics inhibit nerve conduction by reducing the permeability of the neuronal membrane to sodium. This prevents sodium influx which is required for propagation of action potentials.

Lidocaine

PHARMACOKINETICS	ADVERSE EFFECTS	ORDER OF PARALYSIS	NOTES
IV. Little dependence on kidney (<20%) for elimination; dosage adjustment necessary in liver impairment.	Usually cardiac stable, but induces severe tachycardia, bradycardia, A-V block or CHF complications in 1% of patients.	1. Small muscles (fingers, eyes). 2. Limbs, neck, trunk. 3. Intercostal muscles, diaphragm.	Very little histamine release.
IV. Metabolism: Hoffman degradation (breaks ester linkage) in bloodstream.	Moderate histamine release (vasodilation, hypotension).	" "	Administer slowly to avoid massive histamine release.
IV. 80% Hoffman degradation.	Bradycardia, hypotension	" "	
IV. Depends on kidney (60–80%) for elimination; Renal and liver impairment requires dosage adjustments.	Vagolytic (↑ heart rate).	" "	Histamine release is rare.
IV. Cleared by the liver.	Transient hypotension and hypertension		
" "	" "	" "	
IM/IV. Diffuses away from endplate, hydrolyzed by plasma pseudocholinesterase and acetylcholinesterase.	↑ intraocular pressure (contraindicated: open eye wounds) and gastric pressure (caution: reflux during intubation), dysrhythmias. Postoperative muscle pain (myoglobin release and hyperkalemia). May trigger malignant hyperthermia.	1. Fasciculations in chest and abdomen 2. Neck, arms, legs 3. Facial, pharynx, larynx 4. Respiratory muscles	Effects not reversed by acetylcholinesterase inhibitors. Numerous contraindications (e.g., hyperkalemia, burns, digoxin, myopathies, pseudocholinesterase deficiency, glaucoma).

Chemistry: Lidocaine and procaine are the prototype local anesthetics (Table 2.9). All local anesthetics are composed of a hydrophilic domain connected to a hydrophobic domain by an alkyl chain. The drugs are classified as amides or esters according to the type of bond between the hydrophobic domain and the alkyl chain.

Bicarbonate as an adjunct in local anesthesia: Bicarbonate may be added to local anesthetic preparations to increase the percent of anesthetic in the nonionized form. This accelerates penetration of the nerve sheath.

Procaine

Table 2.9 Local Anesthetics, Injectable

DRUG	MECHANISM/ACTIONS	INDICATIONS	UNDESIRABLE EFFECTS
Amides			
Lidocaine (Xylocaine)	Ionized form of drug temporarily reduces the permeability of neuronal membranes to sodium. Thus, action potentials cannot be generated or propagated.	All types of injection and topical anesthesia, sedation, arrhythmias (Table 4.7A), intracranial hypertension.	Drowsiness, dizziness, heart block, arrhythmias, hypotension, myocardial depression.
Ropivacaine (Naropin)	" "	For production of local or regional anesthesia for surgery, post-op pain and obstetrical procedures.	Anxiety
Bupivacaine (Marcaine) (Sensorcaine)	" "	Local infiltration, lumbar, subarachnoid, caudal, peripheral nerve, dental block. Long duration increases utility for epidural block during labor.	Similar to lidocaine. IV administration may induce ventricular arrhythmias.
Mepivacaine (Carbocaine) (Polocaine) (Isocaine)	" "	Infiltration, nerve block, and epidural anesthesia, dental infiltration.	Less drowsiness and amnesia than lidocaine.
Prilocaine (Citanest)	" "	Local anesthesia by nerve block or infiltration in dental procedures.	See Lidocaine; methemoglobinemia in large doses.
Esters			
Procaine (Novocaine)	" "	Low potency. Infiltration and spinal anesthesia.	Low toxicity.
Chloroprocaine (Nesacaine)	" "	Low potency. Infiltration, nerve block, epidural anesthesia.	PERMANENT neural damage may result from use of this agent for spinal anesthesia.
Tetracaine (Pontocaine)	" "	High potency. Spinal anesthesia.	Most toxic ester.

Once internalized, the drug re-equilibrates to the cationic (active) form.

Preferential blockade of small nerve fibers: Pain and temperature fibers (Aδ and C fibers) are more easily penetrated by local anesthetics than larger neurons. The order of loss of nerve function is pain, temperature, touch, proprioception and skeletal muscle tone.

Epinephrine as an adjunct in local anesthesia: Vasoconstriction response to epinephrine causes local hemostasis, inhibiting distribution of local anesthetic away from the site of injection, decreasing systemic absorption and prolonging duration of action at the site of injection.

Consequences of IV injection: When injecting local anesthetics subcutaneously or intramuscularly, aspirate prior to injection to decrease the likelihood of intravascular injection. Systemic absorption can affect the cardiovascular system and the CNS. IV injection is characterized by oral numbness, light headedness, altered taste, or tinnitus. Epinephrine, if included in the anesthetic preparation, will cause transient tachycardia.

ONSET	DURATION	PHARMACOKINETICS	NOTES
Rapid (< 1.5 min) Epidural (5–15 min)	Moderate (few hours)	Metabolized by mixed function oxidases in liver. Some metabolites are active. Excreted in the urine.	Most frequently used.
Rapid (1–5 min) Epidural (15–30 min)	Moderate-long	" "	
Slow (5 min) Epidural (10–20 min)	Long (several hours)	" "	Used when long duration is desired.
Rapid Epidural (5–15 min)	Moderate	" "	Use with caution in renal impairment.
Rapid (<2 minutes) Epidural (5–15 min)	Short		
Rapid Epidural (15–25)	Short (15–60 min)	Metabolized by plasma cholinesterase. Metabolite, *p*-aminobenzoic acid may cause hypersensitivity.	
Moderate Epidural (5–15 min)	Short (30–90 min)	" "	Preferred for those susceptible to malignant hyperthermia.
Slow Epidural (20–30 min)	Moderate	" "	Motor blockade lasts longer than sensory

Chapter 3 **Central Nervous System**

Thousands of neuronal signals race through our brains each moment, controlling our breathing, movements, thoughts and emotions with admirable precision. Neuronal circuits provide the basic "road map" for brain signals, and chemical neurotransmitters carry information from one neuron to another. Neurotransmission in the brain parallels that in the autonomic nervous system (Chapter 2), but utilizes several chemicals and peptides in addition to acetylcholine and norepinephrine. Neurotransmitters that have been most carefully studied are introduced below.

Treatable neurotransmission diseases fall into two categories: those caused by too much neurotransmission and those caused by too little neurotransmission. "Too much" neurotransmission may be due to:

- a focus of hyperexcitable neurons that fire in the absence of appropriate stimuli (e.g., seizure disorders). Therapy is directed toward reducing the automaticity of these cells.

- too many neurotransmitter molecules binding to postsynaptic receptors (possible explanation for psychoses). Therapy includes administration of antagonists which block postsynaptic receptors.

"Too little" neurotransmission may be due to:

- too few neurotransmitter molecules binding to postsynaptic receptors (e.g., depression, Parkinson's disease). Several treatment strategies increase neurotransmission, including 1) drugs that cause release of neurotransmitter stores from the presynaptic terminal, 2) neurotransmitter precursors that are

taken-up into presynaptic neurons and metabolized into active neurotransmitter molecules, 3) drugs which inhibit the enzymes that degrade neurotransmitters and 4) agonists that act at postsynaptic receptors.

Because numerous pathways in the brain use the same neurotransmitter, manipulating transmission in a diseased pathway simultaneously affects synapses of normal neurons. For this reason, CNS drugs are notorious for causing a variety of side effects.

This chapter presents CNS agents according to diseases that are treated by neurotransmission modulators. General anesthetics are also included in this CNS drug chapter, but their mechanism of action does not appear to be mediated by neurotransmitter receptors.

Neurotransmitters of the Brain
• *Norepinephrine*

The synthesis, release and degradation of norepinephrine are presented in Figure 2.4A. Four classes of adrenergic receptors (α_1, α_2, β_1 and β_2) are presented in Table 2.2. Pathways in the brain that utilize norepinephrine have not been clearly identified. Drugs that mimic or modulate norepinephrine transmission are presented in Tables 2.1 to 2.4.

A leading hypothesis suggests that *depression* is caused by impaired monoamine (e.g., norepinephrine, dopamine, serotonin) neurotransmission. Drugs which induce monoamine release are indicated for *attention deficit disorder* and *narcolepsy*.

The biochemical disturbance responsible for these two diseases is unknown.

• *Dopamine*

Dopamine is synthesized from Dopa, the hydroxylated congener of the amino acid tyrosine (Fig. 2.4A). It is degraded by monoamine oxidase A in the brain and monoamine oxidase B outside the CNS and by catechol-O-methyl transferase (COMT).

Dopamine receptors are classified as D_1 or D_2 receptors. Both subtypes reside in numerous regions of the brain. No specific D_1 agonists have been identified. Apomorphine is a D_2 agonist. Activation of either subtype *inhibits* the rate of neuronal firing. Particularly important dopaminergic pathways include 1) the nigrostriatal pathway (from substantia nigra to striatum), 2) neurons of the chemoreceptor trigger zone of the medulla, which controls vomiting, and 3) projections from the hypothalamus to the intermediate lobe of the pituitary, which are thought to regulate prolactin release.

Antipsychotic drugs (Tables 3.3A and 3.3B) inhibit dopamine-stimulated adenylate cyclase (usually associated with D_1 receptor activation) and block D_2 dopamine receptors, suggesting that *psychoses* may result from overstimulation of dopamine receptors. Another disorder, *Parkinson's Disease*, is caused by too little dopaminergic input from the substantia nigra into the striatum. Loss of the nigrostriatal dopamine neurons results in a relative decrease in dopamine input (inhibitory) compared to acetylcholine input (excitatory, Fig. 3.3).

• *5-Hydroxytryptamine (5-HT, Serotonin)*

The amino acid tryptophan is hydroxylated and then decarboxylated to form 5-HT. In neurons, 5-HT is stored (in vesicles), released, taken up into presynaptic neurons and either recycled or metabolized.

5-HT is released from *inhibitory* neurons originating in the raphe nuclei of the pons and midbrain. 5-HT stimulates either 5-HT_1 or 5-HT_2 receptors which are distinguished by the specific antagonist ketanserin (5-HT_2-specific). The hallucinogenic drug, lysergic acid diethylamide (LSD) is a potent agonist at both receptor subtypes. In addition to its role as a neurotransmitter, 5-HT increases small intestine motility and modulates vasodilation. Ninety percent of the body's 5-HT is stored in enterochromaffin cells of the small intestine.

Depression, *attention deficit disorder* and *headaches* have been attributed to serotonergic imbalances. Many serotonergic agents have been developed in the last few years for the treatment of these diseases.

• *Acetylcholine*

The synthesis, release and degradation of acetylcholine are presented in Figure 2.4B. Acetylcholine binds to both muscarinic and nicotinic receptors throughout the brain. Drugs which mimic or modify acetylcholine neurotransmission are presented in Tables 2.5 to 2.9.

A cholinergic antagonist is used in the treatment of Parkinson's disease to correct the imbalance of acetylcholine and dopamine neurotransmission created by the degradation of dopaminergic nerves (Table 3.5). **Rivastigmine**, a cholinergic drug, is used in the symptomatic treatment of Alzheimer's disease. Cholinergic or anti-cholinergic drugs are not otherwise used to treat CNS disorders.

• *Gamma-amino butyric acid (GABA)*

GABA is an *inhibitory* amino acid neurotransmitter of brain interneurons and other cerebral neurons. The enzyme glutamic acid decarboxylase catalyzes the synthesis of GABA from glutamate. GABA is stored in presynaptic vesicles and binds to either GABA-A or GABA-B receptors upon release.

GABA receptors reside on two subunits of a four-subunit receptor complex that surrounds and regulates a chloride ion channel. GABA activation of the receptor induces chloride influx into the neuron. This hyperpolarizes the neuron, making it more difficult to fire when stimulated by excitatory neurotransmitters. Benzodiazepines enhance the actions of GABA at GABA-A receptors, but not GABA-B receptors.

Agents which enhance the actions of GABA such as benzodiazepines and barbiturates are used to treat *anxiety* and *seizures* and as *sedatives* or *muscle relaxants*.

• *Excitatory Amino Acids (EAA)*

Glutamate or a structurally-similar chemical is an *excitatory* neurotransmitter in many areas of the brain. Stimulation of EAA receptors increases cation conductance, leading to depolarization, or stimulates phosphatidyl inositol turnover.

Excitatory amino acids such as glutamate are thought to be important in learning, memory and other brain functions. Glutamate-induced excitotoxicity is implicated in the pathogenesis of Alzheimer's Disease, Huntington's Disease, stroke, epilepsy and amyotrophic lateral sclerosis (ALS). **Riluzole** (Rilutek®), protects neurons from glutamate toxicity in animals and minimally slows progression of ALS.

• *The Opioids*

Endorphins, enkephalins and dynorphins are opiate receptor agonists that are cleaved from a protein called pro-opiomelanocortin. Opiate receptors are located along the periaqueductal gray matter and other brain areas. Morphine and related drugs act at opiate receptors to relieve pain (Table 3.7A, 3.7B). In times of stress or pain, endogenous peptides act at opiate receptors.

• Other Neuropeptides

In addition to the endogenous opiate peptides, several other peptides function as neurotransmitters (e.g., substance P, vasoactive intestinal peptide). These agents are generally cleaved from larger peptide precursors. They can assume a variety of three dimensional shapes, making it difficult to assess the chemistry of peptide-receptor interactions. For this reason, no chemical agonists (other than morphine) or antagonists have been identified for peptide receptors.

Antidepressants

Major depression is characterized by intense sadness or loss of interest in usual activities, accompanied by poor appetite, insomnia or hypersomnia, psychomotor agitation or retardation, decrease in sexual drive, fatigue, feelings of worthlessness, decreased concentration, or thoughts of death or suicide.

Mania, another affective disorder, is characterized by elevated, expansive, or irritable mood, accompanied by increased activity, pressure of speech, flight of ideas, grandiosity, decreased need for sleep, distractibility, or

Table 3.1 Antidepressants

DRUG	MECHANISM/ACTIONS	INDICATIONS	UNDESIRABLE EFFECTS
Tricyclic Antidepressants			
Generally	Not yet clear. Most block reuptake of monoamine neurotransmitters, increasing synaptic levels of the transmitter. Subsequent downregulation (reduction in the number of receptors) of post-synaptic receptors may be the true mechanism of action (Fig. 3.1).	Used to treat major depressive episodes. Also enuresis, agoraphobia (fear of open spaces) with panic attacks, obsessive compulsive neurosis, chronic pain, neuralgia, migraine headaches.	Anticholinergic effects, cardiotoxicity, sedation, orthostatic hypotension, mania, hypomania, weight gain, impotence, obstructive jaundice.
Amitriptyline (Elavil)	" "	Often prescribed by nonpsychiatrists for the disorders listed above.	Most severe anticholinergic effects. Highly sedating.
Imipramine (Tofranil)	" "	Original TCAD. Prescribed less often because of side effects. Enuresis in children.	Less sedating than amitryptiline. Significant anticholinergic effects. Has quinidine-like action that may induce arrhythmias.
Doxepin (Sinequan)	" "	Commonly used for indications described above.	Very sedating, substantial anticholinergic effects.
Desipramine (Norpramin)		Fewer anticholinergic effects.	Less sedation, fewer anticholinergic effects. Sudden death in children has occurred.
Nortriptyline (Pamelor, Aventyl)	" "	Clear relationship between plasma levels and clinical efficacy	Both anticholinergic and sedating.
Amoxapine (Asendin)	" "	Depression.	Moderate anticholinergic and sedative effects. Neuroleptic malignant syndrome.
Protriptyline (Vivactil)	" "	See generally	Least sedation, some anticholinergic effects.
Clomipramine (Anafranil)	" " Very effective serotonin-uptake blocker.	Obsessive compulsive disorder.	Very sedating.
Trimipramine (Surmontil)	" "	Depression	Very sedating.
Monoamine Oxidase Inhibitors			
Tranylcypromine (Parnate) **Isocarboxazid** (Marplan) **Phenelzine** (Nardil) **Selegiline** (Emsam)	Blocks metabolism of biogenic amines (norepinephrine, serotonin, dopamine) increasing the synaptic concentration of these transmitters. Suppresses REM sleep.	Used to treat depression if tricyclic antidepressants fail and when electroconvulsive therapy fails or is refused. Also used to treat narcolepsy, phobic/anxiety states and Parkinson's disease.	Hepatotoxicity, excessive CNS stimulation, orthostatic hypotension. Overdose may cause agitation, hallucinations, hyperreflexia, hyperpyrexia, convulsions, altered blood pressure.

involvement in activities that have high potential for painful consequences. Patients that cycle between depression and mania carry the diagnosis of **bipolar affective disorder.**

The biogenic amine hypothesis suggests that depression is due to paucity of norepinephrine, dopamine, or serotonin neurotransmission in the brain whereas mania is caused by excessive monoamine neurotransmission. The observation that antidepressants increase the synaptic concentration of the monoamines circumstantially supports the biogenic amine hypothesis (Tables 3.1A, 3.1B). Lack of correlation between the onset of drug action (hours) and clinical response (weeks) however, draws criticism to the theory. The latency of antidepressant effects prompted the suggestion that relief from depression may be due to postsynaptic receptor downregulation (expression of fewer receptors at the synaptic membrane) in response to elevated concentrations of biogenic amines that result during antidepressant therapy (Fig. 3.1).

PHARMACOKINETICS	ABUSE POTENTIAL	DRUG INTERACTIONS	NOTES
Well absorbed, widely distributed, highly bound to plasma proteins, half-lives range from 8 hrs to 90 hrs, metabolized more rapidly by children and more slowly by elderly patients.	Tolerance to anticholinergic side effects may develop. Physical and psychic dependence develops occasionally. Sudden withdrawal leads to malaise, chills, coryza and muscle aches.	Do not administer to patients with monoamine oxidase inhibitors in their system (potentiation may be lethal). Other drugs which bind to plasma proteins may displace TCADs. May potentiate effects of other CNS depressants. Potentiate actions of other anticholinergic drugs.	May shorten the cycle length between mania and depression in patients with bipolar disease. Patients coming out of depression are at increased risk of committing suicide because they regain the energy to fulfill their ideations.
PO/IM. Half-life 30–45 hrs	" "	" "	" "
PO/IM. See "generally" above. Half-life 10–25 hrs	" "	" "	" "
PO. " "	" "	" "	" "
" "	" "	" "	" "
" " Half-life 18–45 hrs	" "	" "	" "
" " Shortest half-life 8 hrs	" "	" "	
PO. Longest half-life (75–90 hrs). Thus lower daily dose than other tricyclics.	" "	" "	
See "Generally" above. Half-life 20–35 hrs	" "	" "	
Half-life 7–30 hrs	" "	" "	

Core structure of tricyclic antidepressants

PO. Binds irreversibly to MAO causing pharmacologic effects for weeks. It is inactivated by acetylation. Thus patients who are genetically "slow acetylators" will have elevated serum levels.	Low likelihood of abuse.	Potentiate the effects of sympathomimetics (including tyramine present in dairy and yeast products, amphetamines in diet pills, and sympathomimetics in cold remedies).	Amphetamine-like structure.

Table 3.1 Antidepressants (continued)

DRUG	MECHANISM/ACTIONS	INDICATIONS	UNDESIRABLE EFFECTS
Selective Serotonin Uptake Inhibitors			
Fluoxetine (Prozac)	Selective serotonin reuptake inhibitor (SSRI)	Depression. Obsessive compulsive disorder, bulimia nervosa.	Drug discontinued in 15% of patients due to nausea, headache, nervousness, isomnia, anxiety or diarrhea, altered platelet function; rash.
Sertraline (Zoloft)	" "	Depression, obsessive compulsive disorder, panic disorder.	Nausea, headache, diarrhea, dry mouth, dizziness, insomnia, fatigue, impotence, altered platelet function.
Fluvoxamine (Luvox)	" "	Obsessive compulsive disorder.	Nausea, dry mouth, asthenia.
Paroxetine (Paxil)	" "	Depression, Obsessive compulsive disorder, panic disorder.	Nausea, vomiting, somnolence, insomnia, dizziness, agitation, anxiety, weakness, headache, abnormal ejaculation, altered platelet function.
Citalopram (Celexa) **Escitalopram** (Lexapro)		Depression	
Trazodone (Desyrel)	" "	Depression. Used by some to treat aggressive disorders and cocaine withdrawal.	Rash, hypertension, tachycardia, shortness of breath, many CNS effects reported, ↓ appetite, priaprism.
Vortioxetine (Brintellix)	SSRI and 5-HT3, 5-HT1D, and 5-HT7 antagonist, a 5-HT1A agonist, and a 5-HT1B partial agonist.	Major depressive disorder	Nausea, headache, dry mouth, and dizziness. Suicide risk, worsening depression.
Serotonin-Norepinephrine Uptake Inhibitors			
Venlafaxine (Effexor) **Desvenlafaxine** (Pristiq)	Inhibit serotonin and norepinephrine uptake.	Depression, anxiety.	Sustained hypertension photosensitivity.
Duloxetine (Cymbalta)	" "	Depression, diabetic neuropathic pain.	Hepatotoxicity, sexual dysfunction
Milnacipran (Savella)	" "	Fibromyalgia, depression.	Suicide risk, serotonin syndrome hypertension
Levomilnacipran (Fetzima)	" "	" "	" "
Others			
Mirtazapine (Remeron)	Unknown	Depression, anxiety associated with depression	Low anticholinergic effects, orthostatic hypotension, sedation, agranulocytosis.
Alprazolam (Xanax)	Benzodiazepine with anxiolytic activity. Mechanism of antidepressant effects unknown.	Adjunct to tricyclic antidepressants for depression and panic attacks.	No anticholinergic effects. Does cause sedation and lethargy.
Bupropion (Wellbutrin)	Unknown mechanism.	Depression, smoking cessation.	Seizures, hepatotoxicity, agitation, anticholinergic effects, tremor, nausea, vomiting, headaches.

PHARMACOKINETICS	ABUSE POTENTIAL	DRUG INTERACTIONS	NOTES
Half-life is 48–72 hrs, thus one dose/day. Takes weeks to achieve equilibrium blood levels.		Life-threatening reaction possible with monoamine oxidase inhibitors (MAOI) and with cisapride. Do not use within 2 weeks.	Increased suicide rate reported in patients taking fluoxetine.
PO. Once daily dosing. High plasma protein binding.		MAOI interaction. Similar to fluoxetine. Does not affect levels of other protein-bound drugs.	
PO. Reduce dose with liver dysfunction.		Contraindicated with cisapride.	
PO. Once daily dosing. Reduce dose with hepatic/renal insufficiency.		" " Cimetidine increases paroxetine. Paroxetine reduces phenytoin & digoxin and increases warfarin.	
PO. Well absorbed, extensively metabolized. Effects seen in 1–3 weeks.		Substrate for cytochrome CYP206	
PO. 98% plasma protein binding.		SNRIs, SSRIs, TCAs, triptans, MAOIs, linezolid, meperidine, fentanyl, pentazocine, lithium, tramadol, and antipsychotic agents	
PO. 2–3 doses/day. Reduce w/renal or hepatic problems. Active metabolite is O-desmethylvenlafaxine		" " Substrate for cytochrome CYP2D6	
PO		Substrate CYP2D6 and 1A2.	
PO		Contraindicated with monoamine oxidase inhibitors. Minimal CYP450 metabolism.	
" "			
PO; half-life 20–40 hrs; Extensively metabolized by the liver.		A substrate for cytochrome P450 2D6, 1A2, 3A4.	Tetracyclic structure.
PO. 70% protein bound, half-life = 11 hrs. More rapid onset than tricyclic antidepressants.	Alprazolam has high dependency/abuse potential and a severe withdrawal syndrome.	Few interactions. Additive with other CNS depressants.	
PO. Active metabolites may accumulate, worse w/liver or kidney disease.		Drugs which lower seizure threshold. Bupropion induces P450 enzymes, altering drug metabolism.	Aminoketone structure.

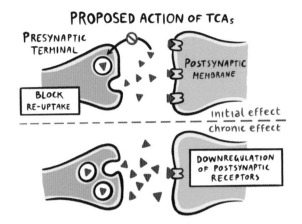

PROPOSED ACTION OF TCAs

PRESYNAPTIC TERMINAL

BLOCK RE-UPTAKE

POSTSYNAPTIC MEMBRANE

Initial effect

chronic effect

DOWNREGULATION OF POSTSYNAPTIC RECEPTORS

Figure 3.1 Possible mechanism of tricyclic antidepressant action. Depression may be due to a relative decrease in monoaminergic neurotransmission. In animal studies, tricyclic antidepressants initially block re-uptake of monoamines, resulting in higher neuro-transmitter concentrations in the synaptic cleft. Over a period of time, the postsynaptic neuron responds to the chronic elevation of monoamines by expressing fewer receptors on the postsynaptic membrane. If indeed clinical response is due to receptor downregulation, then the hypothesis that depression is due to inadequate monoaminergic transmission would be unsatisfactory. It is unclear whether these mechanisms are responsible for relief from depression in humans.

Table 3.2 Central Nervous System (CNS) Stimulants

DRUG	MECHANISM/ACTIONS	INDICATIONS	UNDESIRABLE EFFECTS
Amphetamine-like drugs			
d-Amphetamine (Adderall) **Methylphenidate** (Ritalin) **Dexmethylphenidate** (Focalin)	Releases biogenic amines (NE, dopamine, serotonin) from storage vesicles. CNS stimulant, decreases appetite, improves ability of trained athletes and coordination and performance of fatigued subjects, increases blood pressure.	Narcolepsy, attention deficit disorder in children. No longer recommended for obesity.	CNS overstimulation, restlessness, dizziness, insomnia, increased blood pressure, arrhythmia, anorexia, psychotic episodes.
Non-amphetamine stimulants			
Modafinil (Provigil) **Armodafinil** (Nuvigil)	Inhibit the reuptake of dopamine by binding to the dopamine-reuptake pump	Excessive daytime sleepiness	Headache, rapid heartbeat, skin issues, paresthesias.
Norepinephrine uptake inhibitors			
Atomoxetine (Strattera)	Selectively inhibits norepinephrine uptake.	Attention deficit disorder.	Suicide risk, serious cardiovascular effects, heart rate increase
Narcolepsy Drugs			
Oxybate (Xyrem)	Not yet known	Narcolepsy with cataplexy or excessive daytime sleepiness	Agitation, dizziness, nausea, abnormal thinking, anxiety.
Pitolisant (Wakix)	Blocks H3 autoreceptors to increase histamine at the synapse	Narcolepsy excessive daytime sleepiness	Headache, insomnia, nausea
Methylated Xanthines			
Caffeine	Adenosine receptor antagonist. High dose: ↑ Ca^{++} permeability in sarcoplasmic reticulum and ↑ cAMP by inhibiting phosphodiesterase. Stimulates CNS, constricts cerebral arterioles, induces diuresis, stimulates heart, bronchodilates.	Prolonged apnea in pre-term infants (unlabeled use). Included in some over-the counter analgesic preps, particularly headache remedies.	Insomnia, restlessness, anxiety neurosis, nausea, tachycardia, diuresis.
Theophylline	Cellular mech like caffeine. More CNS stimulation than caffeine. Increased cardiac stimulation and diuresis. More effective bronchodilator.	Bronchial asthma. Apnea and bradycardia in premature infants (unlabeled use).	" "

Why are CNS stimulants prescribed to hyperkinetic children? "Stimulant" is perhaps a misnomer for the actions of amphetamine-like drugs. Although the drugs were first characterized with regard for their ability to stimulate CNS functions, the effects of these drugs are actually very complex. In animal studies, amphetamines accelerate behavior which is slow in the absence of drug and suppress rapid behavior patterns. It has been hypothesized that the sedative effects of amphetamines in hyperkinetic children are due to inhibition of "fast-rate" behavior, and that amphetamine-induced acceleration of "slow-rate" behavior in children with attention deficit disorder may account for improved learning and memory skills.

CNS Stimulants

Attention deficit disorder (ADD) in children is characterized by short attention span, restlessness, distractibility, impulsivity and emotional lability. Hyperactivity is sometimes associated. Amphetamine-like drugs reduce these symptoms in >80% of affected children (Table 3.2). Many treatment plans also involve family counseling and/or psychotherapy. Therapy is usually tailored around the school schedule, the goal being to enhance school performance and encourage behavior which is suitable for the classroom. Drug therapy is often discontinued during school vacations.

PHARMACOKINETICS	TOLERANCE/DEPENDENCE	DRUG INTERACTIONS	NOTES
PO. Well absorbed, enters CNS, excreted without undergoing metabolism, half-life = 4–6 hrs. Elimination is slowed by alkalination of urine.	Often abused. Severe tolerance and dependence. Methamphetamine ("Speed") acts similarly, but is *very* addictive and often abused.	MAO inhibitors: hypertensive crisis, CNS overstimulation, Barbiturates: supraadditive mood elevation. Tricyclic Antidepressants: potentiate CNS stimulation, inhibit metabolism of amphetamine.	Overdose treatment: Acidify urine. Give chlorpromazine to treat CNS symptoms and alpha-receptor blocker to lower blood pressure.
PO. Armodafinil has a longer half-life	" "	Many	Much milder stimulant than amphetamine.
PO. Enters CNS.	Low abuse potential	MAO inhibitors (see amphetamine above)	
PO	Patients using alcohol or benzodiazepines.	Many	
PO		Many	
PO/IM/IV. Rapid complete absorption. Cross placenta, Liver metab. half-life = 3–7 hrs.	Tolerance and dependence likely. Withdrawal may cause headache, anxiety and muscle tension.	Oral contraceptives and cimetidine: inhibit metabolism. Smoking enhances elimination.	85 mg caffeine/cup coffee, 50 mg/cup of tea or cola
PO. half-life = 3.5 hrs in children, 8.5 hrs in adults.	" "	" "	Use decreasing due to toxicity and questionable efficacy.

The anorectic property (appetite suppression) of d-amphetamine may cause growth retardation. These effects are less pronounced with other psychomotor stimulants. Insomnia and nervousness are common side effects of all psychomotor stimulants.

Amongst the methylated xanthines (Table 3.2), caffeine is included in some analgesic preparations because of its CNS-stimulating and cerebrovascular-constricting effects. Many people consume coffee or soft drinks, which contain caffeine, to maintain alertness and to stay awake.

Caffeine is psychologically addicting and tolerance develops to CNS and cardiovascular effects. Withdrawal often results in headaches.

Theophylline is a methylated xanthine which exemplifies a clinically useful drug with a narrow margin of safety. Theophylline is used to treat bronchial asthma as well as apnea and bradycardia in premature infants.

Serum concentrations must be maintained between 10 and 20 µg/ml because it is ineffective at lower concentrations and it produces undesirable effects at higher concentrations.

Antipsychotic Drugs
• Treatment of psychoses

Psychotic Disorders are clinical syndromes characterized by impaired sense of reality, disturbances of thought & emotion, hallucinations (often auditory-"the voice tells me . . . "), delusions ("I possess the power to . . . "), and confusion. The biochemical defects for these diseases have not been clearly elucidated. The syndromes listed may represent several discrete diseases which have similar clinical presentation.

Schizophrenia is a psychotic disorder in which the patient exhibits symptoms listed above for at least six

Table 3.3A Antipsychotic Drugs

DRUG	MECHANISM/ACTIONS	INDICATIONS	UNDESIRABLE EFFECTS
Phenothiazines			
Chlorpromazine (Thorazine) **Thioridazine** **Fluphenazine** (Prolixin) **Perphenazine** **Prochlorperazine** (Compazine) **Trifluoperazine** (Stelazine)	The actions of antipsychotic drugs are complex. The ability of antipsychotics to block D_2 dopamine receptors correlates with their clinical efficacy. Animal studies have shown that dopamine synthesis and metabolism increase with acute treatment and receptor upregulation occurs after a few weeks of antipsychotic administration. It is likely that these effects occur as a regulatory response to the drug-induced decrease in dopaminergic transmission.	Psychoses, including mania, acute idiopathic psychoses and acute episodes of schizophrenia; nausea and vomiting; hiccoughs.	Acute dystonia (abnormal muscle tone), Parkinsonism, malignant syndrome, akathisia, tardive dyskinesia, jaundice, sedation, orthostatic hypotension, anticholinergic effects, adrenergic blocking effects and allergic reactions to the drug. Decreased release of corticotropin and gonadotropins. Increased prolactin secretion. Fewer extrapyramidal symptoms and adrenergic blocking effects than chlorpromazine. More anticholinergic effects. Retrograde ejaculation, decreased testosterone, retinopathy. Less orthostatic hypotension and adrenergic blockade, but more extrapyramidal signs.
Atypical Antipsychotics (fewer extrapyramidal side effects, more effective for treating negative symptoms of schizophrenia)			
Aripiprazole (Abilify) **Brexpiprazole** (Rexulti)	Partial agonist at dopamine D2 and serotonin 5HT1A, receptor antagonist at 5HT2A receptor.	Schizophrenia, mania, depression, autism.	Headache, somnolence, extrapyramidal disorder. Elderly patients with dementia-related psychosis face increased risk of death.
Cariprazine (Vraylar)	Partial agonist at dopamine D2 and D3 receptors	Schizophrenia	Elderly patients with dementia-related psychosis face increased risk of death. Cerebrovascular events, tardive dyskinesia.
Asenapine (Saphris) **Lurasidone** (Latuda)	Unknown	Psychosis, bipolar mania	Somnolence, insomnia, extrapyramidal disorder. Elderly patients with dementia-related psychosis face increased risk of death.
Ziprasidone (Geodon) **Lurasidone** (Latuda)	Unknown. Possible Dopamine D2 and Serotonin 5HT2 antagonist.	Schizophrenia.	Prolonged QT/QTc interval. Risk for arrhythmia and sudden death. Elderly patients with dementia-related psychosis face increased risk of death. Tardive dyskinesia. Somnolence.
Pimavanserin (Nuplazid)	Serotonin 5HT2 antagonist	Psychoses associated with Parkinson's disease.	Elderly patients with dementia-related psychosis face increased risk of death.

months leading to impaired ability to maintain interpersonal relationships, a job, or daily living skills. Active psychosis often occurs only during a small portion of the patient's life. Between psychotic episodes, the patient is often withdrawn and perhaps antisocial.

Widely accepted theories suggest that psychosis is due, at least in part, to excessive dopamine neurotransmission. This theory was originally based on the observation that all antipsychotic drugs blocked D_2 dopamine receptors. More recently, investigators demonstrated that antipsychotic drugs inhibit dopamine-stimulated cAMP production. This action cannot easily be attributed to receptor blockade because dopamine-stimulated cAMP production is linked to D_1 rather than D_2 receptors and antipsychotic drugs have low affinity for D_1 receptors.

• Undesirable Neurologic Effects

As described in the chapter introduction, dopamine is the neurotransmitter of numerous pathways in the brain. Because antipsychotic drugs block *all* D_2 dopamine receptors, they suppress all D_2 receptor-mediated dopamine actions in the brain. Specific neurologic side effects of antipsychotic drugs include:

- **Acute dystonia:** Patients may develop face, neck and back spasms within a week of therapy initiation. Antiparkinsonian drugs reduce symptoms (Table 3.5).
- **Parkinsonism:** Symptoms include "pill-rolling" with fingers, limb rigidity, shuffling gait, bradykinesia, and mask facies caused by dopamine receptor antagonism in the nigrostriatal pathway. Symptoms develop

PHARMACOKINETICS	TOLERANCE/DEPENDENCE	DRUG INTERACTIONS	NOTES
All PO. Chorpromazine and Perphenazine also IM/IV.	Not addicting. Some physical dependence may occur. Tolerance develops to sedative effects. Some cross tolerance, but drugs are not easity substituted for one another. Choreoathetosis may develop upon abrupt withdrawal.	Chlorpromazine enhances the effects of central depressants, sedatives, analgesics, antihistamines, alcohol and morphine. Increases respiratory depression caused by meperidine. Inhibits actions of levodopa and dopamine agonists.	These drugs are sometimes called neuroleptics because they reduce initiative and interest in the environment, alleviate aggressive and impulsive behavior, and reduce spontaneous movement and complex behavior in animals. Generally antipsychotic drugs with more anticholinergic effects produce fewer extrapyramidal side effects.
PO. Well-absorbed.		Many drug interactions.	
PO		Many drug interactions.	
PO. Rapidly absorbed.		" "	
PO.	Low risk of abuse	Drugs that inhibit CYP3A4 activity.	
PO	Low risk of abuse	Many drug interactions.	

within one month of initiating therapy. Parkinsonism is treated with drugs described in Table 3.5.

- **Malignant syndrome:** This relatively rare, but sometimes fatal syndrome is marked by catatonia, rigidity, stupor, fluctuating blood pressure, fever and dysarthria. Antipsychotic drug must be discontinued promptly. Malignant syndrome is treated with bromocriptine (dopamine agonist) or dantrolene (mechanism of action associated with reversing malignant syndrome is unknown), but not antiparkinsonian agents.

- **Akathisia:** Motor restlessness occurring within two months of antipsychotic drug initiation. Decrease dose or discontinue drug. Treat with benzodiazepines or low-dose propranolol.

- **Tardive dyskinesia:** Up to 20% of patients treated with antipsychotics for months to years (particularly phenothiazines and haloperidol) develop involuntary movements of the face, trunk, and extremities (dyskinesia & choreoathetosis). Often non-reversible.

Antiemetics

Dopamine stimulation of D_2 receptors in the chemoreceptor trigger zone (CTZ) of the medulla mediates some forms of nausea and vomiting. Several antipsychotic agents antagonize D_2 receptors in the CTZ, suppressing nausea and vomiting due to cancer chemotherapy agents and other drugs and radiation therapy (Table 3.4). Dopamine antagonists are not the only class of drugs employed to prevent or treat nausea and vomiting. Sero-

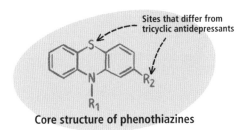

Core structure of phenothiazines

Table 3.3B Antipsychotic Drugs (cont.)

DRUG	MECHANISM/ACTIONS	INDICATIONS	UNDESIRABLE EFFECTS
Miscellaneous			
Clozapine (Clozaril)	Antipsychotic mechanism unclear. Blocks dopamine receptors as well as cholinergic, adrenergic, serotonergic & histaminergic neurotransmission.	Schizophrenia in those whom traditional antipsychotics have failed or have produced intolerable side effects.	Very few extrapyramidal side effects (EPS). Potent antimuscarinic effects. Agranulocytosis in 2%. No tardive dyskinesia or increased prolactin release.
Olanzapine (Zyprexa)	" "	Psychoses.	" "; No agranulocytosis.
Quetiapine (Seroquel)	Higher affinity for 5 HT_2 receptors than D_2 receptors.	Psychoses.	No anticholinergic effects, orthostatic hypotension, sedation; less EPS
Haloperidol (Haldol)	Similar to phenothiazines.	Psychoses, *Tourette's* syndrome, severe behavioral problems in children, hyperactive children (short term), *Huntington's Disease*.	Less sedation, anticholinergic effects, and alpha-adrenergic blocking effects than chlorpromazine. Rarely hypotension. Extrapyramidal side effects may be dramatic.
Pimozide (Orap)	Blocks dopamine receptors.	*Tourette's Syndrome.*	Extrapyramidal disorder, tardive dyskinesia, sedation, headache, sensory changes, hypotension.
Risperidone (Risperdal)	Mechanism unknown. Binds as antagonist at serotonin, dopamine, alpha adrenergic and H1 histamine receptors.	Psychosis.	Extrapyramidal disorder, tardive dyskinesia, sedation, hyperkinesia, somnolence, constipation.
Palilperidone (Invega Sustenna) **Iloperidone** (Fanapt)	Unknown. Possible Dopamine D2 and Serotonin 5HT2 antagonist.	Schizophrenia	Prolonged QT/QTc interval. Elderly patients with dementia-related psychosis face increased risk of death. Dizziness, somnolence, tachycardia, orthostatic hypotension

Table 3.4 Antiemetic/Antivertigo Drugs

DRUG	REMARKS
Prochlorperazine (Compazine)	Prochlorperazine, triflupromazine, chlorpromazine and trifluoperazine are phenothiazine antipsychotics which are described in Table 3.3. These agents control vomiting by blocking D_2 dopamine receptors in the chemoreceptor trigger zone (CTZ) of the brainstem.
Promethazine (Phenergan)	Both a D_2 dopamine antagonist and an H_1 histamine antagonist which is used to control motion sickness as well as nausea and vomiting. Particularly useful following surgery because it reduces anesthesia-related nausea, induces light sleep and reduces apprehension.
Metoclopramide (Reglan)	Dopamine (D_2) antagonist which is particularly useful for reducing chemotherapy-induced nausea. Also used clinically as a GI stimulant to improve gastric emptying. Risk of tardive dyskinesia.
Scopolamine (Transderm-Scop)	This anticholinergic is available as a transdermal preparation to prevent motion sickness. Overdose may cause confusion, memory alterations and other anticholinergic effects.
Anticholinergics/ Antihistamines	Diphenhydramine, dimenhydrinate and meclizine are antihistamines with anticholinergic effects. Anticholinergic drugs reduce motion sickness as well as emesis.
Ondansetron (Zofran) **Granisetron** (Kytril) **Dolastetron** (Anzemet) **Palanosetron** (Aloxi)	Blocks serotonin (5-HT_3) receptors, but not dopamine receptors. Used to control chemotherapy-induced nausea. Remarkably more effective than other agents in patients receiving chemotherapy.

PHARMACOKINETICS	TOLERANCE/DEPENDENCE	DRUG INTERACTIONS	NOTES
PO. Rapid absorption, extensive metabolism.	Abrupt withdrawal may induce psychosis.	Potentiates antihypertensive and anticholinergic agents. Displaces drugs from plasma proteins.	Therapy is with held if granulocyte count is <1500/mm³.
PO	" "	Substrate for P450 isoenzyme CYP1A2	
PO; extensively metabolized in the liver.		Hepatic enzyme inducers and inducers of P450 3A.	
PO/IM/IV. Begin treatment at low dose, individualize dose for each patient.	Transient dyskinesias may be caused by abrupt withdrawal.	Enhances actions of CNS depressants, alcohol, & anticonvulsants. Decreases actions of amphetamines. Severe hypotension with alcohol, epinephrine, antihypertensives. Antimuscarinics: Increase intraocular pressure and reduce haloperidol effects. Lithium: encephalopathic syndrome.	
PO. Serum level does not correlate with activity.	Withdraw slowly. Dyskinesia may develop after abrupt withdrawal.	Lowers seizure threshold in patients taking seizure medications. Potentiates CNS depressants.	
PO. Metabolites active. Reduce dose with liver or kidney dysfunction and in elderly patients.	Withdraw slowly.	Metabolized by P450 enzyme that is inhibited by many other drugs.	Metabolism varies genetically among patients.
PO.	Low risk of abuse.	QT interval-prolonging drugs, Abiraterone, antihypertensives, CYP2D6 or CYP3A4 inhibitors.	

Table 3.5 Drugs Used to Treat Parkinson's Disease

DRUG	MECHANISM/ACTIONS	INDICATIONS	UNDESIRABLE EFFECTS
Levodopa (e.g., I-dopa) Combination products with carbidopa include: Parcopa, Rytary, Sinemet.	Decarboxylated to dopamine (DA) in brain. Improves neurological, motor, and altered mood symptoms of Parkinson's Disease.	Parkinson's disease.	Nausea, vomiting due to stimulation of emetic center (tolerance develops to GI effects), modest orthostatic hypotension, arrhythmias in older patients, involuntary movements (dose limiting), psychiatric disturbances, ↑ sexual activity due to actions on hypothalamus.
Carbidopa (Lodosyn)	Diminishes decarboxylation of I-dopa in peripheral tissues. Improve effect of I-dopa, decreased required dose of I-dopa by about 75%	Used in conjunction with levodopa for Parkinson's disease.	Reduces levodopa-induced nausea and vomiting. Does not alleviate most side effects caused by levodopa. Has no known toxicities when administered alone.
Amantadine (Symmetrel)	Releases DA from intact terminals.	Less effective than I-dopa for treating Parkinson's Disease. Also used to treat drug-induced extrapyramidal reactions.	Few side effects. At high doses may induce hallucinations, confusion & nightmares.
Ergot-derivative dopamine receptor agonists			
Bromocriptine (Parlodel)	Powerful D_2 agonist.	Parkinson's disease, particularly when tolerance develops to I-dopa or when symptom relief "swings" between doses. Also hyperprolactinemia, adjunct in treatment of pituitary tumors.	More nausea, hallucinations, confusion, and hypotension than I-dopa. Less dyskinesia. Nonspecific CNS arousal.
Nonergot-derivative dopamine receptor agonists			
Rotigotine (Neupro)	Dopamine receptor agonist.	Parkinson's Disease, Restless leg syndrome.	Somnolence, hallucinations, psychoses, hypotension, impulse control deficits.
Pramipexole (Mirapex)	" "	" "	" "
Monamine oxidase inhibitors			
Selegilene (Eldepryl) **Rasagiline** (Azilect) **Safinamide** (Xadago)	Irreversibly inhibits monoamine oxidase type B (but not type A). Inhibits intracerebral metabolic degradation of DA.	Parkinson's disease as adjunct to levodopa and carbidopa.	" "
Catechol-O-methyltransferase (COMT) inhibitors			
Entacapone (Comtan) **Tolcapone** (Tasmar)	Selective, reversible COMT inhibitor	" "	" "
Anticholinergic drugs (also listed in Table 2.7)			
Trihexyphenidyl (Artane) **Biperiden (**Akineton) **Benztropine** (Cogentin)	Antagonists at cholinergic receptors. Lessen ACh:DA imbalance in striatum. Less effective than I-dopa for tremor and other symptoms.	" "	" "

PHARMACOKINETICS	DRUG INTERACTIONS	NOTES
PO. Rapidly absorbed, half-life = 1–3 hrs. Less than 1% of levodopa penetrates CNS because of peripheral decarboxylation. This is circumvented by coadministration of carbidopa, a dopa decarboxylase inhibitor.	Pyridoxine: may reduce effects of levodopa by stimulating decarboxylation. Antipsychotic drugs: block DA receptors. MAO inhibitors: cause buildup of sympathomimetic amines (withdraw 2 weeks before administration of levodopa). Anticholinergic drugs: synergism with levodopa, may delay absorption by slowing gastric emptying. Antidepressant drugs: ↑ orthostatic hypotension.	Rarely used without coadministration of dopa decarboxylase inhibitors (carbidopa).
PO. Pills contain fixed amounts of carbidopa and levodopa (Sinemet).		Has no pharmacological action when given alone.
PO. Must adjust dose with renal failure	Anticholinergic agents: Enhance CNS side effects.	Less effective than l-dopa, more effective than anticholinergics. Also an antiviral drug (Table 7.11).
PO. Initiate at low dose and individualize. Rapid, partial absorption. Half-life = 1.5–3 hrs.	May be used with l-dopa/carbidopa	
Transdermal patch	Few interactions.	
PO	" "	
PO. Rapidly absorbed. Crosses blood brain barrier. Metabolized in liver.	Potentiates effects of sympathomimetics	Slows progression of Parkinson's when used in conjunction with levodopa/carbidopa.
PO	Drugs metabolized by COMT. MAO inhibitors.	
PO	" "	

tonin (5-HT$_3$) antagonists are potent antiemetics, particularly useful for chemotherapy-induced nausea. A few cholinergic antagonists and histamine antagonists reduce emesis and control motion sickness (Table 3.4). The neural pathways influenced by these antagonists have not been clearly identified.

Anti-Parkinson Drugs

Parkinson's Disease affects a half million Americans. Symptoms include tremor (pill-rolling) at rest, bradykinesia (slow movements), and cogwheel rigidity.

The disease is caused by decreased dopamine neurotransmission in the nigrostriatal pathway secondary to degradation of dopaminergic neurons that project from the substantia nigra to the striatum (caudate and putamen). Figures 3.2 and 3.3 outline the neuropathology of Parkinson's Disease. Treatment consists of either increasing dopamine neurotransmission or blocking cholinergic neurotransmission (Table 3.5, Fig. 3.3).

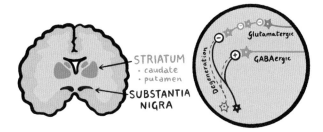

Figure 3.2 The symptoms of Parkinson's Disease are caused by degeneration of dopaminergic neurons in the nigrostriatal pathway. Inhibitory dopaminergic neurons which project from the substantia nigra to the caudate and putamen are most affected. Cholinergic input (excitatory) to the caudate and putamen appears to be unaffected; thus the balance is tipped toward cholinergic input.

Movement Disorder Drugs

Tardive dyskinesia is a serious side effect of antipsychotic medications that manifests as repetitive jerking movements of the tongue, face and neck. For many pa-

Table 3.6A Opioid Analgesics and Antagonists

DRUG	MECHANISM/ACTIONS	INDICATIONS	UNDESIRABLE EFFECTS
Full Agonists			
Morphine	Opiate receptor agonist. Induces analgesia, sedation, respiratory depression, nausea, vomiting, vertigo, miosis, ADH release, GI effects (decreased propulsion and secretions, tonic spasm). Increases tone in bile duct, bronchi, ureters, and bladder.	Severe pain which cannot be alleviated by non-narcotic analgesics or weaker narcotic analgesics. Drug of choice for treating severe pain of myocardial infarction.	Respiratory depression, constipation, CNS disturbances, orthostatic hypotension, cholestasis, nausea and vomiting with initial doses.
Levorphanol (Levo-dromoran) Oxymorphone Oxycodone (Oxycontin) Hydromorphone (Dilaudid) Tramadol (Ultram) Hydrocodone (Vicodin)	" "	Moderate to severe pain.	" "
Meperidine (Demerol)	" "	Also used to treat rigors such as those induced by amphotericin B.	Like morphine. Overdose causes convulsions due to excitatory actions of metabolite.
Methadone	Full morphine-like actions, weaker sedative.	Detoxification of narcotic addiction. Severe pain in hospitalized patients.	Similar to morphine.
Fentanyl (Sublimaze)	More potent than morphine.	Preoperative medication used in anesthesia.	Muscle rigidity, bradycardia.
Sufentanil	Potent analgesic.	Used in anesthesia.	Little data available.
Alfentanil	See Fentanyl.	" "	" "
Remifentanil (Ultiva)	" "	" "	May cause chest wall rigidity if infused rapidly.

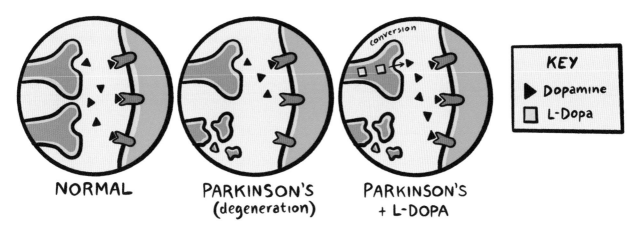

Figure 3.3 Synaptic view of Parkinson's Disease (PD) and therapy. *Dopaminergic terminals decay in PD, leading to decreased dopamine (DA, solid triangles). L-dopa, an amino acid precursor of DA crosses the blood brain barrier, enters surviving DA terminals and is converted to DA. Increased DA neurotransmission partially restores the dopamine-acetylcholine neurotransmission balance.*

NORMAL   PARKINSON'S (degeneration)   PARKINSON'S + L-DOPA

KEY
▶ Dopamine
☐ L-Dopa

tients, discontinuing the medication that causes tardive dyskinesia is not a good option because they rely on the medicine for mental health. **Valbenazine tosylate** (Ingrezza) and **Deutetrabenazine** (Austedo) are vesicular monoamine transporter 2 (VMAT2) inhibitors that reduce the movement symptoms of tardive dyskinesia.

PHARMACOKINETIC	TOLERANCE/DEPENDENCE	DRUG INTERACTIONS	NOTES
IM/PO/PR/SC/IV, epidural, intrathecal. Poorly absorbed, metabolized by conjugation w/glucuronic acid. 4–6 hr duration.	Tolerance develops to analgesic effects, but not to constipating effects. High abuse potential. Withdrawal leads to insomnia, pain, increased GI activity, restlessness.	Enhances actions of other CNS depressants. Increases neuromuscular blocker-induced respiratory depression. Additive with drugs that cause hypotension.	The analgesic actions of opioids are threefold. The perception of pain is reduced (increased threshold), the unpleasant psychological response is reduced, and sleep is induced even in the presence of pain.
Various. Better oral absorption than morphine.	" "	" "	" "
IM/SC/PO/IV. Shorter duration than morphine. Metabolite is excitatory to CNS.	" "	With MAO inhibitors, causes severe CNS excitation, respiratory depression, or hypotension.	" "
IM/SC/PO. Excreted more slowly than morphine (half-life = 25 h). Withdrawal symptoms are less intense, but prolonged.	Cross dependent with morphine (basis for narcotic detoxification). Tolerance develops readily. Less psychologically addicting than morphine.		Detoxification replaces heroin dependence with methadone dependence. Then slowly reducing methadone dose to zero.
IV. Rapid onset. Half-life = 4 h. Shorter duration than morphine.			Transdermal, transmucosal preparation available for chronic pain.
IV, sublingual	Little data available.		
IV. Fastest onset.	" "		
IV.	" "		IV tubing must be changed or cleared after remifentanil.

Huntington's disease (HD) is a neurodegenerative and movement disorder caused by an expansion of the triplet repeat "CAG" in the huntingtin gene. Deutetrabenazine (described immediately above) is also indicated for reducing the choreic movements of HD. Depression and suicide are risks of this drug in HD patients. Xenazine (tetrabenazine) is the first medication FDA has approved specifically for Huntington's. Like Deutetrabenazine, it is a VMAT2 inhibitor. It helps suppress jerky involuntary movements, but it may cause serious side effects, such as worsening depression.

Drugs to Treat Alzheimer's

Alzheimer's disease (AD) is the most common type of dementia. AD is thought to be caused by the abnormal build-up of proteins in and around brain cells. One of the proteins involved is called amyloid, deposits of which form plaques around brain cells. The other protein is called tau, deposits of which form tangles within brain cells. AD is a disease that progresses from mild to profound memory loss and diminished ability to converse or interact with the environment. AD involves parts of the brain that control thought, memory, and language. FDA approved drugs to treat Alzheimer's include two categories.

Monoclonal antibodies such as Lecanemab (Leqembi) and Aducanumab (Aduhelm) reduce beta amyloid plaques and are indicated for patients with mild disease. Donepezil (Aricept®), Rivastigmine (Exelon®), and Galantamine (Razadyne®) are drugs that inhibit the acetylcholinesterase enzyme, which normally breaks down acetylcholine. The main pharmacological actions of these drugs are believed to occur as the result of this enzyme inhibition, enhancing cholinergic transmission, which relieves the symptoms of Alzheimer's dementia.

Drugs to Treat ALS

Amyotrophic lateral sclerosis (ALS) is an uncommon neurologic disorder that involves degeneration of the motor neurons that control voluntary muscle movement. As the disease progresses, individuals have increasing difficulty chewing, swallowing, walking, talking, and ultimately breathing. Onset of symptoms is typically between age 40 and age 70 and patients typically survive 2-10 years after diagnosis. In 8-23% of patients, the disorder is caused by a heritable mutation in the superoxide dismutase 1 (SOD1) gene. In others, no genetic defects can be identified. The FDA approved Tofersen (Qalsody) to treat patients with amyotrophic lateral sclerosis (ALS)

Table 3.6B Opioid Analgesics and Antagonist (cont.)

DRUG	MECHANISM/ACTIONS	INDICATIONS	UNDESIRABLE EFFECTS
Weak Agonists			
Codeine	A prodrug: 10% of dose is converted to morphine. Actions are due to morphine. Also an antitussive (suppresses coughing).	Minor pain relief. Cough.	Similar to morphine, but less intense at doses which relieve moderate pain. At high doses, toxicity is as severe as with morphine.
Mixed Agonist-antagonists—lower abuse potential			
Buprenorphine	In contrast to full opioid agonists, buprenorphine is a partial agonist that does not cause the euphoric high.	Moderate to severe pain. Preoperative medicine, combination anesthesia.	Respiratory depression, sedation, dizziness, nausea, vomiting.
Pure Antagonists			
Naloxone (Narcan)	Surmountably blocks opioid receptors. Has no effect in narcotic-free persons.	Treatment of narcotic overdose. Diagnostic agent (for evaluation of addiction) in methadone programs. To reduce postoperative respiratory depression.	Induces narcotic withdrawal syndrome (appetite loss, muscle contraction, fever/chills, restlessness, cardiovascular and respiratory symptoms, nausea, vomiting, diarrhea.)
Naltrexone (ReVia)	Similar to naloxone, but longer duration.	" ". Also indicated for treatment of alcoholism.	" "

associated with a mutation in the superoxide dismutase 1 (SOD1) gene (SOD1-ALS). Tofersen is an antisense oligonucleotide that targets SOD1 mRNA to reduce the synthesis of SOD1 protein. The approval was based on a reduction in plasma neurofilament light (NfL), a blood-based biomarker of axonal (nerve) injury and neurodegeneration. Tofersen is administered intrathecally (through a spinal injection) by healthcare professionals. This drug is not approved for patients who lack a mutation in the SOD1 gene. **Edaravone** (Radicava) is an anti-oxidant that may scavenge oxygen free radicals and slow the progression of ALS. **Riluzole** (Rilutek, Tiglutik, Excervan) inhibits glutamate release and extends the life of ALS patients by about 3 months.

Central Analgesics
• The Opioid System

Opium, derived from poppies, relieves pain and induces euphoria by binding to "opiate receptors" in the brain. These opioid drugs mimic the actions of three peptide families in the brain known as the endorphins, the enkephalins, and the dynorphins. These peptides, along with several nonopioid peptides (MSH, ACTH, & lipotropin) are cleaved from the protein precursors pro-opiomelanocortin (POMC), proenkephalin, and prodynorphin (Fig. 3.4).

Three subtypes of receptors, mu, kappa and delta, mediate the effects of opioid drugs and peptides. The prototype agonist is morphine, which is a potent analgesic and sedative. Agonists with similar analgesic effects (full agonists) are described in Table 3.6A and partial agonists are described in Table 3.6B. Opioid agonists also reduce intestinal motility (antidiarrheals), reduce coughing (antitussives) and induce vomiting. Nonanalgesic agonists used for these purposes are listed in Table 3.6C.

Patients on morphine and related agonists must be monitored for signs of CNS-mediated respiratory depression, which is the dose-limiting side effect of opioid agonists.

Principles that should be kept in mind when prescribing pain relievers include:

- Narcotic analgesics should be employed only when pain cannot be relieved by non-narcotic analgesics (Chapter 9).
- Abuse and street-sales of narcotic agents are common. Monitor patients for drug-seeking behavior.
- Remind patients that constipation is a likely side effect and that a stool softener may be necessary.

PHARMACOKINETICS	TOLERANCE/DEPENDENCE	DRUG INTERACTIONS	NOTES
PO/SC/IM. Rapid absorption, half-life = 3 h. 10% demethylated to form morphine, the rest is conjugated in liver and excreted in urine.	Low risk of abuse.	Similar to morphine.	Included in a number of cough medicine preparations because of antitussive effects.
Various.	Abstinence syndrome upon withdrawal. Lower abuse potential than morphine.	Increase CNS depression caused by CNS depressants.	Antagonist activity: - Bupromorphine > Butorphanol > Desocine = Nalbuphine > Pentazocine.
IV. Rapid onset, short half-life (< 1 h).	Induces abstinence syndrome in narcotic-dependent patients.	Reverses narcotic-induced depression.	
PO. Duration > 24 h.	" "	" "	

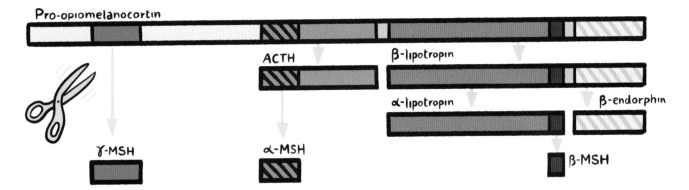

Figure 3.4 Cleavage of **pro-opiomelanocortin (POMC)** *into β-endorphin and non-opioid peptides.* *POMC serves as a precursor (pro-) for the opiate peptide, β-endorphin (-opio-); for α-, β- and γ-melanocyte-stimulating hormone (MSH, -melano-); for adrenocorticotrophic hormone (ACTH, -cort-); and for α- and β- lipotropin (-in). Notice that the peptides are not located end-to-end, but that some of the smaller peptide sequences are embedded in larger sequences (e.g., α-lipotropin, β-MSH and β-endorphin are contained within β-lipotropin). Two other protein precursors contain enkephalins and dynorphins.* **Proenkephalin** *contains seven met-enkephalin sequences (Tyr-Gly-Gly-Phe-Met).* **Prodynorphin** *contains three leu-enkephalin sequences (Tyr-Gly-Gly-Phe-Leu) and the sequences for dynorphin A, Dynorphin B, α-neodymorphin and β-neoendorphin.*

Table 3.6C Nonanalgesic Uses of Opioids

DRUG	REMARKS
Diphenoxylate	Diphenoxylate is used to treat diarrhea. It is too insoluble to escape the GI tract. Like morphine, it causes constipation, but diphenoxylate fails to produce analgesia. Antidiarrheal effects can be blocked by narcotic antagonists.
Dextromethorphan	Dextromethorphan is the dextro- isomer of codeine. It is included in cough medicine because of its centrally acting antitussive effects. Dextromethorphan actions are unaffected by narcotic antagonists. It causes little sedation or GI disturbances.
Apomorphine	Stimulates the chemoreceptor trigger zone, causing nausea and vomiting. These emetic effects are blocked by narcotic antagonists. Apomorphine has few other narcotic-like effects. Sublingual form of apomorphine is now approved for Parkinson's disease.

Anti-anxiety Agents

Barbiturates and benzodiazepines enhance the actions of the inhibitory neurotransmitter, gamma-aminobutyric acid (Fig 3.5, Tables 3.8A, 3.8B and 3.8C). Agents from both classes are effective sedative-hypnotics (sleep-inducing agents), antianxiety agents, and anticonvulsants (Table 3.9). Benzodiazepines are prescribed more often than barbiturates because they cause fewer side effects.

Flumazenil (Romazicon) is a competitive antagonist at benzodiazepine receptors. Used clinically to reverse benzodiazepine sedation or overdose and as part of the treatment for hepatic encephalopathy. Resedation occurs in about 10% of reversals. Seizures infrequently occur with reversal, usually following multi-drug overdose.

Anticonvulsants

Seizures occur as a result of hyperactivity or hyper-synchronicity of neurons in the brain. Focal seizures

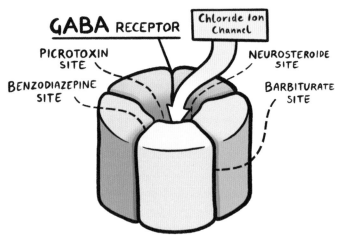

Figure 3.5. Schematic model of the GABA/Benzodiazepine/Barbiturate receptor complex. *The receptor complex surrounds a chloride ion channel. Gamma-amino butyric acid (GABA) is an inhibitory neurotransmitter. GABA binds to the receptor causing chloride influx. The movement of chloride into the neuron hyperpolarizes the neuronal membrane, making it more difficult for excitatory neurotransmitters to depolarize the cell. Benzodiazepines and barbiturates enhance the actions of GABA, but fail to open the chloride channel in the absence of GABA.*

Table 3.8A Comparison of Benzodiazepines and Barbiturates

BARBITURATES	BENZODIAZEPINES
Mechanism/Actions: Bind to receptor adjacent to GABA receptor on chloride channels. Results in retention of GABA at its receptor causing increased flux of chloride through the channel. Induces sedation, euphoria, other mood alterations, hypnosis, "barbiturate" fast waves in EEG, respiratory depression. At high doses, may cause cardiovascular depression or death.	**Mechanism/Actions:** Bind to benzodiazepine site on neuronal GABA receptor complex. Enhances GABA-mediated chloride influx (neuronal inhibition). At therapeutic doses may also inhibit neurons by unknown mechanisms which are unrelated to either GABA or chloride influx. Cause sedation, skeletal muscle relaxation, and "barbiturate" fast waves on EEG. Also has anticonvulsant effects.
Indications: Clinical uses include treatment of epileptic seizures and as a component of anesthesia. Benzodiazepines are usually preferred to barbiturates for treatment of anxiety. Antipsychotics are preferred for treatment of neurotic states.	**Indications:** Generally, benzodiazepines are used for treatment of anxiety and neurotic states, nervous tension, agitation, psychosomatic illness, delerium tremens. Also used for skeletal muscle relaxant, anticonvulsant, and sedative properties. Diazepam is the benzodiazepine of choice for muscle relaxation and intractable seizures.
Undesirable effects: Drowsiness, clouding of consciousness, dysarthria, ataxia, "paradoxical" stimulation due to behavioral disinhibition, CNS depression to the point of coma and respiratory arrest, laryngospasm.	**Undesirable Effects:** Drowsiness, clouding of consciousness, dysarthria, ataxia, behavioral disinhibition, dermatitis.
Pharmacokinetics: PO/PR/IM/IV. Well absorbed orally. Give IM only if patient can't take orally. Give IV slowly because of hypotension risk. Barbiturates vary markedly in lipid solubility and plasma protein binding (Table 3.8B). Barbiturates induce P450 enzymes in the liver which ↑ metabolism of phenytoin, digitoxin, coumadin and others.	**Pharmacokinetics:** Primary difference between various benzodiazepine agonists are their pharmacokinetic properties (Table 3.8C).
Tolerance/Dependence: Tolerance, metabolic dependence, and psychologic dependence are likely. Dependence presents much like chronic alcoholism. Upon withdrawal, convulsions, hyperthermia, and delerium may be severe enough to cause death.	**Tolerance/Dependence:** High dose, chronic therapy may lead to dependence. Abrupt withdrawal may cause syndrome that mimics alcohol withdrawal (convulsions, hyperthermia, delerium). Cross tolerance and dependence occur.
Drug Interactions: Barbiturates as a class interact with over 40 other drugs. These interactions are largely due to alteration of metabolizing enzymes in the liver or interference with the absorption of other drugs.	**Drug Interactions:** Additive with alcohol.

involve a cluster of neurons and present with unilateral symptoms. They may be due to structural abnormalities such as scars, tumors or inflammation.

Generalized seizures involve both hemispheres. They occur either as a result of hyperexcitability throughout the brain or because an epileptic focus spreads to both sides of the brain. By the latter mechanism, focal seizures may become generalized.

• Types of Seizures and Drugs of Choice

• **Partial Seizures:** *Simple* partial seizures consist of a single detectable motor, sensory or psychological dysfunction which does not change during an episode. Consciousness is retained throughout. Partial *complex* seizures begin in a focal area, usually in the temporal lobe or limbic cortex, and spread. Focal signs are often followed by automatisms (e.g., lip smacking, sweat-

ing) and dulled or lost consciousness. Effective drugs include **carbamazepine, phenytoin, clonazepam and primidone. Valproic acid** is sometimes added.

• **Absence Seizures (Petit mal):** Generalized seizures in children or teens which present as brief episodes of blank staring but no convulsions. Effective drugs include **ethosuximide, valproate, clonazepam and trimethadione**.

• **Generalized Tonic-Clonic Seizures (Grand mal):** Begin with prolonged contractions of muscles in extension followed by cyanosis due to arrested breathing. Patients then experience whole-body clonic jerks. Treatment options include **phenytoin, diazepam carbamazepine, phenobarbital and primidone**.

• **Status Epilepticus:** Continuous series of seizures without reawakening. May cause permanent brain damage. Intravenous, **diazepam, phenytoin** or **phenobarbitol** is recommended for treatment.

Table 3.8B Comparison of Barbiturates

DRUGS	REMARKS
Long Acting Phenobarbital Primidone	Duration: 10–12 hours. Barbital is excreted primarily by the kidneys. Phenobarbital is metabolized by the P450 enzymes in the liver. Phenobarbital induces P450 enzymes, causing increased metabolism of many drugs. Phenobarbital is used clinically as an anticonvulsant.
Short Acting Amobarbital Pentobarbital Secobarbital	Duration: 3–6 hours. Metabolized by P450 enzymes in liver. Amobarbital is sometimes administered by psychiatrists during analysis or therapy. Prior to some neurosurgical procedures (e.g., temporal lobectomy for intractable seizures) amobarbital is injected unilaterally into the carotid artery to determine the dominant hemisphere of the brain.
Ultra-short Acting Methohexital	Duration: <3 hours. These drugs are deposited in fat, then secondarily metabolized by the liver.

Table 3.8C Comparison of Benzodiazepines

DRUG	METABOLISM	NOTES
Long Acting		
Diazepam (Valium)	Most rapidly absorbed. Metabolized in liver to active metabolites which prolong clinical duration of action. Metabolized slowly by infants, elderly and patients with hepatic disease.	Indicated for anxiety disorders.
Quazepam (Doral)	Active metabolites prolong duration of action.	Commonly used for insomnia.
Estazolam (Prosom)	Metabolites are minimally active.	Indicated for insomnia.
Clonazepam (Klonopin)	" "	Used primarily for anxiety disorders.
Chlorazepate (Tranxene)	PRODRUG is hydrolyzed in stomach to active agent.	" "
Chlordiazepoxide (Librium)	Longest duration of action.	" "
Shorter Acting		
Alprazolam (Xanax)	Metabolites not active.	Has antidepressant actions as well as anxiolytic actions. Also used to treat panic attacks. Unlike many benzodiazepines, alprazolam does not cause daytime drowsiness.
Lorazepam (Ativan)	Metabolites not active.	Useful for achieving rapid sedation of agitated patients. No daytime sedation.
Oxazepam (Serax)	Poorly absorbed, requires higher doses than diazepam to achieve same effects.	Useful for treating elderly patients and patients with liver dysfunction because it does not rely on the liver for metabolism.
Temazepam (Restoril)	Metabolites may be active.	
Triazolam (Halcion)		Used for insomnia. Addictive potential.

• *Principles of Anticonvulsant Therapy*

- Increase dose of suitable single agent until desired effect is achieved or until toxicity prevents further increase.

- Follow serum drug levels.

- A second drug may be added if maximal doses of the initial drug fail. The initial drug should then be tapered and discontinued.

- Abrupt discontinuance of an anticonvulsant may induce status epilepticus. Always taper doses.

- Inform female patients of association with birth defects.

General Anesthetics

Inhalation anesthetics are vapors used during surgery to achieve sedation, muscle relaxation and analgesia. The first anesthetic, ether, was introduced in 1846 by a second-year medical student at Massachusetts General Hospital. Ether has since been replaced by non-volatile agents.

Inhalation anesthetics do not appear to work through a receptor mechanism and the mechanism of action remains a mystery. Theories suggesting that anesthetics work by altering the lipids in cell membranes stem from the observation that the potency of anesthetics correlates extremely closely with the solubility of the drug in oil.

Migraine Headache Therapy

Sumatriptan (Imitrex®, Onzetra Xsail, Zembrace Sym-Touch), **naratriptan** (Amerge), **rizatriptan** (Maxalt), **Almotriptan** (Axert), **Elitriptan** (Relpax), **Frovatriptan** (Frova) and **zolmitriptan** (Zomig) are vascular $5HT_1$ (serotonin) receptor agonists that cause vasoconstriction of the basilar artery and dura mater vessels. Pain relief occurs in 15 – 80% of patients. Onset of relief is 10–120 minutes. Toxicity includes; dizziness, tingling, flushing, chest discomfort, weakness, neck pain, and marked hypertension. **Fremanezumab** (Ajovy), **Erenumab** (Aimovig), **Eptinezumab** (Vyepti) and **Galcanezumab** (Emgality) are injectable drugs that block the calcitonin gene-related peptide (CGRP). **Rimegepant** (Nurtec) and **Ubrogepant** (Ubrelvy) are oral CGRP antagonists. Propranolol and timolol are used to prevent onset of migraine headaches (Table 2.4).

Table 3.9 Epilepsy Drugs

DRUG	MECHANISM/ACTIONS	INDICATIONS	UNDESIRABLE EFFECTS
Diazepam (Valium) Lorazepam (Ativan)	Enhances GABA-mediated chloride influx (Fig. 3.6).	Status epilepticus. Rapid onset useful for stopping active seizures. Not used for chronic seizure control.	Drowsiness, clouding of consciousness, ataxia, other signs of CNS depression.
Clonazepam Clorazepate	" "	Alternative to ethosuximide or valproic acid for absence seizure.	" "
Clobazam	" "	Lennox-Gastaut syndrome	" "
Felbamate	NMDA receptor antagonist and GABA potentiation.	Focal seizures, Lennox-Gastaut syndrome	GI distress, nervousness, drowsiness
Tiagabine (Gabitril)	Blocks presynaptic GABA-uptake.	Partial seizures.	Dizziness, nervousness, tremor.
Vigabatrin (Sabril)	Blocks GABA breakdown	Complex partial seizures	Dizziness, dyscoordination
Phenytoin (Dilantin) Fosphenytoin (Cerebyx)	Reduces sodium, calcium and potassium currents across neuronal membranes. Unclear which effects are responsible for seizure prophylaxis.	All types of seizures except absence.	Nystagmus, ataxia, other CNS disturbances, bone marrow suppression, gingival hyperplasia, hepatotoxicity, GI disturbances.
Carbamazepine (Tegretol) Oxcarbazepine (Trileptal) Eslicarbazepine (Aptiom)	Similar to phenytoin. Also has antidiuretic effect. Chemical structure similar to tricyclic antidepressants.	All types of seizures except absence. Trigeminal neuralgia, manic depression, schizophrenia that fails to respond to antipsychotics.	Agranulocytosis or aplastic anemia (monitor blood counts), vertigo, nausea, vomiting.
Valproic Acid (Depakote)	Mechanism unknown. Enhancement of GABA neurotransmission postulated.	All seizure types, particularly disorders of combined seizure types. Manic episodes in bipolar disorder.	Severe/fatal hepatotoxicity, particularly in small children, much less in adults. Thrombocytopenia, hyperammonemia.
Ethosuximide (Zarontin)	Mechanism unknown.	Absence seizures.	Nausea, vomiting, decreased appetite, and weight loss.
Gabapentin (Neurontin)	Mechanism unknown. Related to GABA, but likely acts at distinct receptor.	Adjunctive treatment of partial seizures.	Somnolence, ataxia, dizziness, other CNS effects.
Lamotrigine (Lamictal)	Mechanism unclear. May stabilize neurons and affect glutamate/aspartate release.	Adult patients with partial seizures or Lennox-Gastaut Syndrome.	Dizziness, headache, nausea, ataxia, somnolence, diplopia, blurred vision. Life-threatening rash in children (1:50) and adults (1:1000).
Topiramate (Topamax)	Mechanism unknown. May be related to actions at GABA or kainate/AMPA receptors.	Partial onset seizures.	Psychomotor slowing. Somnolence, ataxia, dizziness, speech impairment.
Zonisamide (Zonegran)	Mechanism unclear. May block sodium channels or facilitate dopamine or serotonin.	" "	Elevated body temperature in some children. Agitation, irritability.
Rufinamide	Inhibits sodium channel.	Lennox-Gastaut Syndrome seizures.	Central nervous system adverse effects.
Levetiracetam (Keppra)	Unknown.	Myoclonic, partial onset, primary generalized.	Somnolence, dizziness, behavioral change.
Levetiracetam (Keppra)	Unknown.	Myoclonic, partial onset, primary generalized.	Somnolence, dizziness, behavioral change.
Pregabalin (Lyrica)	GABA receptor agonist.	Neuropathic pain, seizures, fibromyalgia.	Dizziness, somnolence, headache, blurred vision, weight gain.
Ethosuximide (Zarontin)	Mechanism unknown.	Absence seizures.	Nausea, vomiting, decreased appetite, and weight loss.
Lacosamide (Vimpat)	Enhances slow inactivation of voltage-gated sodium channels.	With other drugs for partial seizures.	Dizziness, nausea, vomiting.
Perampanel		With other drugs for partial seizures.	Dizziness, drowsiness, nausea.
Brivaracetam (Briviact)	Synaptic vesicle protein 2A (SV2A) ligand	Seizure disorders	Suicide risk, neurologic and psychiatric effects

PHARMACOKINETICS	DRUG INTERACTIONS
IV/PO/PR. Rapid onset (IV <5 min). Metabolized in liver. Diazepam has longer half-life.	Additive with CNS depressants. Many drugs inhibit metabolism of diazepam.
PO.	Additive with CNS depressants.
PO.	" "
PO. Acts in 1-4 hours	Other seizure medications
PO. Titrate dose over 6–20 weeks.	Other anticonvulsants
PO/IV/IM. Therapeutic serum level is 10–20 mcg/ml. Slow onset, long half-life. Metabolized in liver.	Many drugs alter metabolism and protein binding of phenytoin and vice-versa.
PO. Induces its own metabolism by stimulating P450 enzymes in liver.	Do not administer to patients with monoamine oxidase inhibitors (Table 3.1B) in their system (potentiation may be lethal).
PO/IV. Metabolized in liver, highly protein bound, half-life longer in children and patients with liver damage.	Additive with other anticonvulsants. Levels decreased by aspirin and cimetidine.
PO. Metabolized in liver, not protein bound. Therapeutic level 40–100 mcg/ml.	Ethosuximide increases phenytoin levels and decreases primidone.
PO. Excreted unchanged by kidneys. Reduce dose w/renal dysfunction.	Gabapentin absorption decreased by antacids.
PO. Induces its own metabolism.	Reduce dose if patient is on valproate. Other anticonvulsants may reduce serum levels.
PO. Excreted unchanged by kidneys. Reduce dose with renal impairment.	Reduces levels (efficacy) of oral contraceptives. Enhances CNS depressants.
PO.	Drugs that reduce liver enzymes ↑ metabolism.
PO.	" "
PO. Rapid absorption.	May cause toxicity with carbamezepine.
PO. Rapid absorption.	May cause toxicity with carbamezepine.
PO. Minimal metabolism.	ACE inhibitors, CNS depressants.
PO. Metabolized in liver, not protein bound. Therapeutic level 40–100 mcg/ml.	Ethosuximide increases phenytoin levels and decreases primidone.
PO. Well absorbed. Food does not affect absorption.	Few interactions.
PO.	
PO.	CYP2C19 inhibitors

Table 3.10 General Anesthetics

DRUG	REMARKS[1]
Thiopental (Pentothal–see Tables 3.8A and B)	**CNS:** Sedation, hypnosis, CNS depression, decreased cerebral blood flow and metabolism (reduced intracranial pressure). **CV:** 10–20% drop in blood pressure. **Resp:** Apnea, bronchoconstriction. **Tox:** Hypotension, tachycardia, resp depression, bronchospasm, anaphylaxis. **Kinetics:** IV. Onset 40 seconds, duration 30 minutes, drug released from fat stores may prolong anesthesia.
Propofol (Diprivan)	**CNS:** More potent than thiopental. **CV:** Bradycardia, hypotension, decreased myocardial perfusion. **Resp:** Apnea. **Tox:** Pain on injection (use lidocaine first), CNS stimulation, severe cardiovascular depression in elderly and hypovolemic patients. **Kinetics:** IV. Onset 1 min. Very rapidly cleared by metabolism and tissue distribution. Constant infusion necessary to maintain anesthesia.
Etomidate (Amidate)	**CNS/CV/Resp:** Similar to thiopental, less cardiovascular and respiratory depression. **Tox:** Myoclonus, vomiting, adrenal insufficiency from chronic use. **Kin:** IV. Onset 1 min, Duration 3–5 min.
Ketamine (Ketalar)	**CNS:** Dissociative (disconnected from surroundings) anesthesia, analgesia, increased intracranial pressure. **CV:** Increase or decrease in blood pressure, heart rate. **Resp:** Apnea, bronchodilation. **Tox:** Hallucinations (Adults > children), nightmares, increased secretions. **Kinetics:** IV/IM. Onset 30 sec, Duration 15 min.
Volatile Organics **-Halothane (H)*** (Fluothane) **-Enflurane (E)*** (Ethrane) **-Isoflurane (I)*** (Forane)	**CNS:** Anesthesia, skeletal muscle relaxation. **CV:** Myocardial depression (*E > H > I), decreased vascular resistance, sensitize heart to catecholamines (*H > E > I). **Resp:** Respiratory depression, bronchodilation (*H > E > I). **Tox:** Malignant hyperthermia possible with all. Halothane associated with hepatotoxicity and infrequent liver failure. Enflurane: nephrotoxicity **Kinetics:** Isoflurane is least metabolized, lack of metabolites credited for hepatic & renal safety. All stored in fat. Newer agents include **Desflurane and Sevoflurane**.
Nitrous Oxide	**CNS:** 100% Nitrous oxide fails to induce anesthesia in >50% of people–usually used with other agents. **CV:** When combined with halothane or enflurane, less hypotension at equivalent depth of anesthesia. **Resp:** Little effect. **Tox:** Transient hypoxia following use. **Kinetics:** Least soluble in blood. Thus, excreted rapidly by expiration of unmetabolized gas.

[1] The molecular mechanism of action is unknown for most anesthetics. Agents often used with an anxiolytic (Table 3.8) and/or paralytic (Table 2.9). Drugs are rapidly distributed, metabolized in the liver and excreted by the kidney unless noted.

Chapter 4 **Cardiovascular and Hematology Drugs**

In simple terms,

- The heart is a **pump**.
- It pumps blood through a system of blood vessels that has a **limited volume capacity**.
- An **electric conduction system** maintains regular rate and rhythm.
- Myocardial cells **require oxygen**.

When heart function is considered in these terms, heart malfunctions and therapeutic interventions can be predicted:

- **Heart failure** occurs when the heart can no longer pump enough blood to meet the metabolic demands of the body. The most common cause is myocardial injury from ischemia, inflammation and chronic hypertension.
- **Hypertension** develops when blood volume is great compared to the space available inside blood vessels. Mean arterial pressure is equal to cardiac output times peripheral resistance. Increased heart rate, decreased vascular resistance and myocardial contractility, enhance cardiac output. Vasoconstriction elevates peripheral resistance.
- **Arrhythmias** occur when electrical signals become irregular.

- **Angina** (chest pain) is the heart's way of signalling that some of its cells are not getting enough oxygen (too little blood flow). **Myocardial infarction** occurs when oxygen-starved areas of the heart begin dying.

An understanding of the pathophysiology of each disease and the therapeutic goals of each treatment strategy will make learning the individual drugs much easier. Table 4.1, which follows, describes the pharmacologic approach to treating heart malfunctions. Note that some drugs are used to treat several malfunctions.

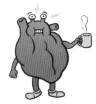

Antihypertensives
• *Diuretics*

Diuretics reduce blood pressure and edema by increasing urine production. All diuretics enhance water and sodium excretion, but the effect of diuretics on other salts depends on the mechanism of action (Table 4.2A, Fig. 4.1).

- **Thiazide diuretics** inhibit sodium and chloride reabsorption in the distal tubule, resulting in mild diuresis. Potassium supplements may be necessary because of potassium-wasting effects.

Table 4.1A Strategies for Treating Cardiovascular Disease

THERAPEUTIC GOALS	PHARMACOLOGIC STRATEGIES Prototype drug listed, alternative drugs listed in following tables

Hypertension

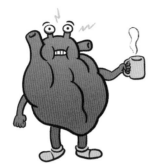

Reduce volume overload

Diuretics decrease blood volume by increasing the volume of water excreted in the urine.

Reduce sympathetic outflow from the brain

Clonidine is an agonist at α_2 receptors. Clonidine inhibits further release of the sympathetic agonist, norepinephrine, and inhibits sympathetic outflow from the brain.

Block adrenergic receptors in the heart

Atenolol is a β_1 adrenergic receptor antagonist that reduces heart rate and myocardial work.

Dilate blood vessels

Prazosin blocks α_1 adrenergic receptors, causing vasodilation.

Nifedipine blocks calcium entry into smooth muscle cells of arterial walls, preventing contraction.

Hydralazine relaxes arterioles.

Captopril reduces production of angiotensin II, causes vasodilation.

Angina

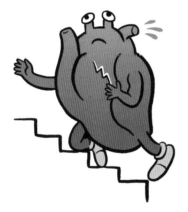

- **Stable Angina**

Nitroglycerin reduces preload by venodilation.

Atenolol decreases myocardial work (β1 antagonist)

Diltiazem decreases blood pressure through vasodilation, by blocking calcium entry, and decreases heart rate, thereby decreasing O_2 demand and consumption.

- **Unstable Angina**

Beta blockers reduce heart rate and myocardial work.

Aspirin prevents platelet aggregation in myocardial arteries.

Heparin inhibits clotting in myocardial arteries.

Nitroglycerin reduces preload.

Eptifibatide or **Tirofiban** inhibit platelet aggregation.

Reduce work of heart and improve cardial circulation

Myocardial Infarction

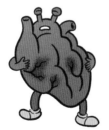

Reperfuse ischemic tissue

Streptokinase converts plasminogen to plasmin. Plasmin digests fibrin and fibrinogen, thus dissolving clots.

Antianginal agents See above. Not nifedipine, which is dangerous in setting of myocardial infarction.

Table 4.1B Strategies for Treating Cardiovascular Disease (cont.)

THERAPEUTIC GOALS	PHARMACOLOGIC STRATEGIES Prototype drug listed, alternative drugs listed in following tables

Heart Failure

Reduce workload.

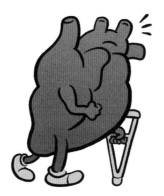

Improve myocardial contractility.

Diuretics decreases blood volume.

Natrecor (Nesiritide), a BNP (Brain Naturetic Peptide) analog causes a naturesis, decreasing preload and improving cardiac contractility.

Captopril causes vasodilation.

Atenolol (β blocker) reduces heart rate and work load.

Nitroglycerin reduces venous tone thereby decreasing preload. (It also dilates coronary arteries, enhancing blood delivery to the heart).

Hydralazine and **Nitroprusside** relax arterioles.

Digoxin increases calcium influx into myocardial cells.

Amrinone inhibits cAMP degradation (cAMP is a biochemical messenger that stimulates the heart).

Dobutamine increases cAMP production by stimulating β_1 adrenergic receptors.

Arrhythmias

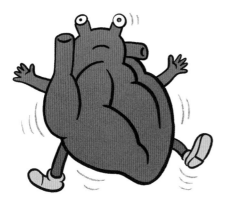

Restore synchronous myocardial contraction

Several classes of agents described in Tables 4.7A & B.

Vascular Occlusion

Prevent coagulation

Warfarin, heparin

Direct thrombin inhibitors (bivalirudin)

Prevent platelet aggregation

Aspirin

Thienopyridines (clopidogrel)

GP IIb/IIIa inhibitors (abciximab)

Destroy clots that have already formed

tPA

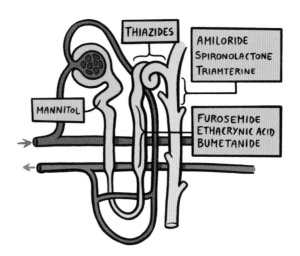

Figure 4.1 Site of diuretic actions. *Thiazide diuretics inhibit sodium and chloride reabsorption in the distal tubule. Loop diuretics inhibit chloride reabsorption in the thick ascending loop of Henle. Potassium sparing diuretics inhibit potassium secretion and influence sodium excretion in the collecting tubule. Mannitol osmotically inhibits water and sodium reabsorption throughout the nephron.*

Table 4.2A Antihypertensive Agents – Diuretics

DRUG	MECHANISM/ACTIONS	INDICATIONS	UNDESIRABLE EFFECTS
Thiazide Diuretics			
Hydrocholorothiazide (Oretic)	Inhibits sodium and chloride reabsorption in the distal tubule. Loss of K^+, Na^+, and Cl^- causes increase in urine output. Sodium loss results in ↓ GFR.	Ideal starting agent for hypertension, chronic edema, idiopathic hypercalcuria.	Hypokalemia, hyponatremia, hyperglycemia, hyperuricemia, hypercalcemia, oliguria, anuria, weakness, decreased placental flow, sulfonamide allergy, GI distress.
Loop Diuretics			
Furosemide (Lasix) **Torsemide** (Soaanz)	Inhibits chloride reabsorption in thick ascending loop of Henle. High loss of K^+ in urine.	Preferred diuretic in patients with low GFR and in hypertensive emergencies. Also, edema, pulmonary edema, and to mobilize large volumes of fluid. Sometimes used to reduce serum potassium levels.	Hyponatremia, hypokalemia, dehydration, hypotension, hyperglycemia, hyperuricemia, hypocalcemia, ototoxicity, sulfonamide allergy, hypomagnesemia, hypochloremic alkalosis, hypovolemia.
Ethacrynic Acid (Ethacrynate)	" "	Orally for edema, IV for pulmonary edema.	Most ototoxic, more GI distress, less likely to cause alkalosis. Otherwise like furosemide.
Bumetanide (Bumex)	Most potent.	Orally for edema, IV for pulmonary edema.	Similar to furosemide. Ototoxicity has not been reported.
Potassium Sparing Diuretics			
Amiloride (Midamor)	Directly increases Na^+ excretion and decreases K^+ secretion in distal convoluted tubule.	Used with other diuretics because K^+-sparing effects lessen hypokalemic effects. May correct metabolic alkalosis.	HYPERkalemia, sodium or water depletion. Patients with diabetes mellitus may develop glucose intolerance.
Spironolactone (e.g., Aldactone)	Antagonist of aldosterone (aldosterone causes Na^+ retention). Also has actions similar to amiloride.	Used with thiazides for edema (in congestive heart failure), cirrhosis, and nephrotic syndrome. Also to treat or diagnose hyperaldosteronism.	As for amiloride. Also causes endocrine imbalances (acne, oily skin, hirsutism, gynecomastia). Less gynecomastia with eplerenone.
Triamterene (Dyrenium)	Directly inhibits Na^+ reabsorption and secretion of K^+ and H^+ in collecting tubule.	Not used for hyperaldosteronism. Otherwise like spironalactone.	May turn urine blue and decrease renal blood flow. Otherwise like amiloride.
Carbonic Anhydrase Inhibitors			
Acetazolamide	Block carbonic anhydrase.	Congestive heart failure.	Acidosis, rash, or other hypersensitivity.
Osmotic Diuretic			
Mannitol	Osmotically inhibits sodium and water reabsorption. Initially increases plasma volume and blood pressure.	Acute renal failure, acute closed angle glaucoma, brain edema, to remove overdoses of some drugs.	Headache, nausea, vomiting, chills, dizziness, polydipsia, lethargy, confusion, and chest pain.

Antihypertensives (cont.)

- **Loop diuretics** are more powerful than thiazides and must be used cautiously to avoid dehydration. These agents may cause hypokalemia, so potassium levels should be followed closely.

- **Potassium-sparing diuretics** enhance sodium and water excretion while retaining potassium. These agents are marketed in combination with potassium-wasted diuretics in order to minimize potassium imbalances.

- **Osmotic diuretics** draw water into the urine, without interfering with ion secretion or absorption in the kidney.

• Antiadrenergics

Andrenergic agonists increase blood pressure by stimulating the heart (β1 receptors) and/or constricting peripheral blood vessels (α1 receptors). In hypertensive patients, adrenergic effects can be suppressed by inhibiting release of adrenergic agonists or by antagonizing adrenergic receptors (Table 4.2B & C).

- **Presynaptic adrenergic release inhibitors** are divided into "central" and "peripheral" antiadrenergics (Table 4.2B). **Central** antiadrenergics prevent sympathetic (adrenergic) outflow from the brain by activating inhibitory α2 receptors. By reducing sympathetic outflow, these agents encourage "parasympathetic predominance". Thus, the list of

PHARMACOKINETICS	CONTRAINDICATIONS	DRUG INTERACTIONS	NOTES
PO. Absorbed rapidly, eliminated primarily as unchanged drug.	Pregnant women (unless clearly indicated for pathologic edema) Anuria.	Increases toxicity of digitalis or lithium; hypokalemia with corticosteroids or ACTH; orthostatic hypotension with alcohol, barbiturates or with narcotics. Decreases effects of vasopressors.	There are many thiazide-like diuretics which differ primarily in dosage requirements and duration. Consult a drug index for these details.
PO/IV. 95% protein bound, eliminated unchanged by kidney. Torsemide is longer acting. PO once daily.	Anuria, electrolyte depletion.	Increases toxicity of ototoxic and nephrotoxic drugs and lithium. Probenecid and indomethacin inhibit diuretic effects of furosemide. Enhances effect of antihypertensive drugs.	Signs of hypochloremic alkalosis include tetany; increased bicarbonate, heart rate BUN, and hematocrit; decreased blood pressure, sodium, and skin turgor.
Similar to furosemide. Narrower dose-response curve than furosemide.	" "		Ethacrynate sodium is used intravenously to treat acute pulmonary edema.
PO/IV. 95% absorbed, 95% protein bound, half metabolized, half-life = 1.5 hrs.	" "		
PO. Excreted unchanged in kidney, 6 hr half-life. Can be used in patients with hepatic insufficiency.		Severe hyperkalemia with potassium supplements. Increased hyperkalemia with other K$^+$-sparing diuretics.	More rapid onset than spironolactone.
PO. Metabolized extensively in liver to an active metabolite. Half-life = 1–1.5 days (4–6 hr. For eplerenone)	Anuria, substantial renal insufficiency, hyperkalemia. Avoid in diabetics.	As for amiloride. Also increases risk of digoxin toxicity and decreases vasopressor action of norepinephrine.	The metabolite canrenone is primarily responsible for the actions of this drug.
PO. Rapidly absorbed, highly metabolized, rapidly excreted.	" "	" "	Marketed in combination with thiazide diuretics.
PO/IV.	Hypersensitivity, acidosis, closed angle glaucoma.	Cyclosporine, salicylates.	Also used for open angle glaucoma.
IV.	Heart failure, hypertension, pulmonary edema because of transient increase in blood pressure.		Initially increases central venous pressure, therefore may induce heart failure in susceptible patients.

undesirable effects resembles the list of parasympathetic actions (Fig 2.3). **Peripheral** antiadrenergics prevent norepinephrine release from peripheral nerve terminals (e.g., those which terminate on the heart). These agents deplete norepinephrine stores in nerve terminals.

- **Alpha and beta blockers** compete with endogenous agonists for adrenergic receptors. Antagonist occupation of α1 receptors inhibits vasoconstriction

and occupation of β1 receptors prevents adrenergic stimulation of the heart.

Selective α1 or β1 blockers are replacing nonspecific β blockers, because they produce fewer undesirable effects. Several β blockers have intrinsic sympathomimetic activity (act as weak agonists at some adrenergic receptors). These drugs stimulate β2 receptors, which reduces the likelihood that rebound hypertension (sympathetic reflex

Table 4.2B Antihypertensive Agents – Presynaptic Adrenergic Release Inhibitors

DRUG	MECHANISM/ACTIONS	INDICATIONS	UNDESIRABLE EFFECTS
Central anti-adrenergics (See Table 2.3)			
Clonidine (Catapres)	Acts in brain as postsynaptic α2-adrenergic agonist causing reduction in sympathetic nervous system activity (decreased heart rate, cardiac ouput and blood pressure). Exact mechanism unknown.	Mild to moderate hypertension.	Rash, drowsiness, dry mouth, constipation, headache, impaired ejaculation. Rebound hypertension if withdrawn abruptly. To limit toxicity, start with low dose and increase slowly.
Methyldopa (Aldomet)	As for clonidine. Also, synthesized to methylnorepinephrine which acts as a weak sympathomimetic "false neurotransmitter" which decreases sympathetic outflow from the CNS.	As for clonidine. Used to treat hypertension in pregnant women.	Dry mouth, sedations, slight orthostatic hypotension. Some patients experience impotence, psychic disturbances, nightmares, involuntary movements, or hepatotoxicity.
Guanabenz (Wytensin) **Guanfacine** (Tenex)	As for clonidine. Also depletes norepinephrine stores in peripheral adrenergic nerve terminals.	Mild to moderate hypertension.	Dry mouth, sedation, Rebound hypertension is observed less frequently.
Peripheral anti-adrenergics (See Table 2.3)			
Reserpine (e.g., Serpasil)	Partially depletes catecholamine stores in peripheral nervous system and perhaps in the CNS. Decreases total peripheral resistance, heart rate, and cardiac output.	Seldom used for mild to moderate hypertension. No longer recommended for psychiatric disorders.	"Parasympathetic predominence" (bradycardia, diarrhea, bronchoconstriction, increased secretions), decreased cardiac contractility and output, postural hypotension (depletes norepinephrine inhibiting vasoconstriction) peptic ulcers, sedation and suicidal depression, impaired ejaculation, gynecomastia. Low risk or rebound hypertension because of long duration of action.
Guanethidine	Sequestered into adrenergic nerve endings. Initially releases norepinephrine (increase BP and HR). Then depletes norepinephrine from terminal and interferes with release.Reflex tachycardia is then impossible because of depletion of norepinephrine.	Severe hypertension *when* other agents fail. *Rarely used.*	Initial increase in heart rate and blood pressure (due to release of norepinephrine). Resting and orthostatic hypotension. Brady-cardia, decreased cardiac output, dyspnea in COPD patients, severe nasal congestion. No depression (poor CNS penetration)
Guanadrel (Hylorel)	Like guanethidine, but works faster, releases norepinephrine initially (transient increase in blood pressure), and has little CNS activity.	Mild to moderate hypertension.	As for guanethidine, but less severe.

to fall in blood pressure) will develop. Activated β2 receptors dilate large central arteries which provide a reservoir for blood.

• *Vasodilators*

The previous table presented drugs that caused vasodilation by blocking α1- mediated vasoconstriction. Vasodilation can also be induced by inhibiting other endogenous vasoconstrictors or by activating a vasodilation pathway (Tables 4.2D & 4.3). Examples of vasodilators include:

• **Angiotensin converting enzyme (ACE) inhibitors** suppress the synthesis of angiotensin II, a potent vasoconstrictor. In addition, ACE inhibitors may induce production of vasodilators in the body.

PHARMACOKINETICS	CONTRAINDICATIONS	DRUG INTERACTIONS	NOTES
PO. Readily absorbed, 75% bioavailability, eliminated largely unchanged by kidney. Must decrease dose w/renal insufficiency.	Hypersensitivity to clonidine.	Tricyclinc antidepressants reduce antihypertensive effects. Alcohol, barbiturates and sedatives increase CNS depression. Concomitant withdrawal of β-blockers ↑ rebound hypertension.	If blood pressure drop is too great, reflex renin production may cause sodium and water retention. Diuretics may counteract this.
PO/IV. Although 63% excreted unchanged by kidneys, it can be used in patients with renal insufficiency.	If signs of heart failure (due to fluid retention as a result of decreased renal blood flow) occur, discontinue drug. Contraindicated in those with liver dysfunction.	Similar to clonidine.	Antibodies to methyldopa may cause hemolytic anemia (fairly rare, but potentially lethal). Follow CBC.
PO. Decrease dose with renal or hepatic dysfunction		Similar to clonidine. Thiazide diuretics increase antihypertensive effects.	
PO. Well absorbed, extensively metabolized. Plasma half-life is shorter than therapeutic half-life, suggesting that drug may be retained at its site of action.	Because of "parasympathetic predominance", contraindicated in patients with congestive heart failure, asthma, bronchitis, peptic ulcer disease. Patients with family history of depression.	Action of direct-acting catecholamines are sharply increased. Reduces effectiveness of mixed or indirect sympathomimetics. Causes severe hypertension with MAO inhibitors. Causes severe bradycardia, heart block or failure with digitalis, quinidine,or beta blockers. Potentiates action of antihypertensive agents or CNS-depressants.	DO NOT administer MAO inhibitors and reserpine within two weeks of each other.
PO. Incompletely absorbed, >30% bioavailability, half eliminated unchanged, half as metabolites. Because of very long half-life (5 days), maximal actions may not develop for 2 weeks.	Patients with pheochromocytoma will experience severe hypertension.	Tricyclic antidepressants inhibit uptake into neuron decreasing antihypertensive effects. Other interactions similar to reserpine (above).	Because of long half-life, effects may persist up to two weeks after discontinuation.
PO. Incompletely absorbed, excreted unchanged (50%) and as metabolites (50%). Shorter half-life (12 hrs) than guanethidine.	" "	" "	

Table 4.2C Antihypertensive Agents – Alpha and Beta Blockers

DRUG	MECHANISM/ACTIONS	INDICATIONS	UNDESIRABLE EFFECTS
α adrenergic antagonists (also described in Table 2.4)			
Prazosin (Minipress) **Terazosin Doxazosin** (Cardura)	Peripheral alpha-1 adrenergic antagonist. Dilates both arteries and veins.	Hypertension and hypertension with congestive heart failure.	Hypotension (postural hypotension on first dose is sudden and severe). Sodium depletion (often caused by diet or diuretic therapy in hypertensive patients) worsens the hypotensive episodes. Edema, dry mouth, congestion, headache, nightmares, sexual dysfunction and lethargy may also be observed.
Mixed α and β antagonists			
Labetalol (e.g., Trandate) **Carvedilol** (Coreg)	Blocks α1, β1 and β2. Achieves lower blood pressure (α1) without reflex tachycardia (β1 blockade).	Hypertension.	Further suppresses failing heart. Fatigue, impotence, diarrhea, numbness, orthostatic hypotension.
β adrenergic antagonists (also described in Table 2.4)			
Atenolol (Tenormin) **Betaxolol** (Kerlone) **Carteolol** (Cartrol) **Penbutolol** (Levatol) **Bisoprolol** (Zebeta)	Preferentially blocks β1 adrenergic receptors. Decreases heart rate and output and ↓ renin release. Less bronchoconstriction than agents which bind to β2 receptors	Good starting therapy for mild to moderate hypertension	Further suppresses failing heart. CNS sedation and depression.
Metoprolol (Lopressor)	" "	" "	" "
Accbutolol (Sectral)	Has some intrinsic sympathomimetic activity as well as β1 blocking activity.	" "	" "
Esmolol (Brevibloc)	Similar to atenolol (no sympathomimetic activity)	Cardiosuppression in acute MI and unstable angina.	" "
Propranolol (e.g., Inderal)	Blocks both β1 and β2 adrenergic receptors. Decreases heart rate and output and ↓ renin release. Bronchoconstriction via antagonism of β2 receptors.	" "	Transient hypertension due to antagonism of β2 receptors (which dilate large arteries) and reflex response to decreased cardiac output, bronchospasm, otherwise like atenolol.
Nadolol (Corgard)	" "	" "	" "
Timolol	" "	" "	" "
Pindolol (Visken)	Has some intrinsic sympathomimetic activity as well as β1 and β2 blocking activity.	" "	Intrinsic sympathomimetic activity *decreases likelihood of rebound hypertension* (by dilating large arteries via β2) or bronchospasm

PHARMACOKINETICS	CONTRAIND.	DRUG INTERACTIONS	NOTES
PO. 50% bioavailability, >90% plasma protein bound, eliminated as unchanged drug and as metabolites. Terazosin, Doxazosin, and Tamsulosin have longer half lives than Prazosin, which permits once daily dosing.		Phenobarbital shortens its half-life. Enhances actions of other antihypertensives, may produce severe hypotension.	Because of severe orthostatic hypotension, patients should be lying down and observed for at least two hours after initial doses.
PO/IM/IV. Well absorbed, high first pass metabolism, metabolized in liver. Reduce Carvedilol dose w/renal or liver dysfunction.	Contraindicated in patients with asthma or bradycardia.	Labetalol: Myocardial depression w/halothane. Blocks β-agonist induced bronchodilation. Carvedilol: Increases effects/toxicity of calcium entry blockers, clonidine, digoxin, insulin, antidiabetics.	
PO. Long half-life allows once/ day dosing. Poor penetration into brain (fewer CNS effects). Excreted unmetabolized. Decrease dose w/renal dysfunction.	Severe diabetes, bradycardia, partial heart block, severe heart failure, asthma, emphysema.	All β blockers may enhance effects of digoxin and lidocaine	
PO. Shorter half-life, metabolized by liver, enters brain.	" "	Levels of metaprolol may be ↑ by verapamil, cimetidine, or oral contraceptives.	
PO. Moderate half-life, administered once-twice/day.	" "	See Atenolol.	
IV. Short duration (half-life = 9 min) because it is metabolized by erythrocyte esterase.	" "	" "	Under investigation for use in hypertensive emergencies.
PO. Good CNS penetration (more severe side effects).	" "	Cimetidine increases serum concentration of propranolol.	Abrupt discontinuation may cause rebound hypertension and tachycardia. Increases risk of stroke, angina, arrhythmias, infarction.
PO. Poor CNS penetration. Decrease dose w/renal dysfunction.	" "	See atenolol.	" "
PO. Longer half-life than propranolol (it is not metabolized). Enters CNS, but causes fewer side effects than propranolol.	" "	" "	" "
PO. Metabolized by liver.	" "		

67

• **Calcium entry blockers** prevent calcium influx into the muscle cells of blood vessel walls. Smooth muscle relies on the influx of extracellular calcium for contraction. Blockade of the calcium influx prevents contraction, causing vasodilation. Smooth muscle is also responsible for propulsion in the GI tract. Inhibition of propulsion by calcium channel blockers causes constipation, a prevalent side effect of calcium channel blocker therapy. Cardiac muscle and conducting tissue rely on rapid influx of sodium and slow influx of calcium through separate channels for contraction. The slow

Table 4.2D Antihypertensive Agents – Vasodilators

DRUG	MECHANISM/ACTIONS	INDICATIONS	UNDESIRABLE EFFECTS
ACE inhibitors			
Captopril (Capoten) **Lisinopril** (e.g., Prinivil) **Enalapril** (Vasotec) **Ramipril** (Altase) **Benazepril** (Lotensin) **Fosinopril** (Monopril) **Moexipril** (Univasc) **Trandolapril** (Mavik) **Perindopril** (Aceon)	Inhibits angiotensin converting enzyme (ACE) in the lung, which reduces synthesis of the vasoconstrictor, angiotensin II. Suppresses aldosterone, resulting in natriuresis. Potentiates other vasodilators (e.g., bradykinin, prostaglandins).	Hypertension. Particularly useful for high-renin hypertension. Preferred drug for hypertensive patients with diabetic nephropathy because glucose levels are not affected. Heart failure – used with diuretics and digitalis. Myocardial infarction – to enhance heart reperfusion.	All ACE inhibitors: First dose hypotension, dizziness, proteinuria, rash, tachycardia, headache, cough. Captopril infrequently causes agranulocytosis or neutropenia.
Angiotensin II antagonists			
Losartan (Cozaar) **Valsartan** **Irbesartan** (Avapro) **Candesartan** (Atacand) **Telmisartan** (Micardis) **Eprosartan** (Teveten) **Olmesartan** (Benicar) **Azilsartan** (Edarbi)	Antagonist at angiotensin II receptor of vascular muscle.	Hypertension	Hypotension, dizziness.
Aldosterone Receptor Antagonists			
Eplerenone (Inspra)	Blocks binding of aldosterone to mineralocorticoid receptor	Hypertension, congestive heart failure post-MI.	Hyperkalemia, nephrotoxicity.
Direct vasodilators			
Hydralazine (Apresoline)	Relaxes arterioles (not veins) independent of sympathetic interactions. Decreases blood pressure leading to reflex tachycardia and increased cardiac output. Directly increases renal blood flow.	Moderate hypertension. May be used in pregnant women who are hypertensive.	Reflex tachycardia, palpitations, fluid retention, systemic lupus erythematosis-like syndrome. Chronic therapy may lead to peripheral neuritis (due to interference with vitamin B6 metabolism in neural tissue).
Minoxidil (Loniten)	" "	Hypertension not controlled by other drugs. Marketed for male pattern baldness.	As for hydralazine. Also, cardiac muscle lesions, pulmonary damage, hirsutism.
Isoxsuprine (Vasodilan)	Skeletal muscle vasodilator.	Peripheral or cerebral vascular insufficiency.	Dizziness, hypotension, tachycardia, GI distress.
Papaverine (e.g., Pavabid)	Smooth muscle dilator. Mechanism not defined.	Peripheral, cerebral and myocardial (with arrhythmias) ischemia.	Tachycardia sedation, GI distress, chronic hepatitis.
Epoprostenal (Flolan)	Pulmonary and systemic arterial vasodilation, ↓ platelet aggregation.	Primary pulmonary hypertension.	Flushing, headache, GI distress, hypotension, jaw pain.
Nitroprusside (Nipride)	Converted to nitric oxide, which induces cGMP. cGMP stimulates a phosphorylation/dephosphorylation cascade. Relaxes smooth muscle by dephosphorylating myosin.	Continuous intravenous infusion used in hypertensive crisis.	Severe hypotension, cyanide toxicity, hepatotoxicity.
Fenoldopam (Corlopam)	Dopamine agonist (D_1 selective)	Used in hypertensive emergencies.	Dose-related fall in BP. Increase in heart rate.

calcium channel is particularly important in the S-A and A-V nodes. Blockade of these channels slows the heart. Skeletal muscle contraction is induced by rapid influx of sodium, which triggers the release of calcium from the sarcoplasmic reticulum. Because these cells do not require extracellular calcium for contraction, calcium channel blockers fail to affect skeletal muscle.

- **Direct Vasodilators** relax smooth muscle cells which surround blood vessels by a mechanism which is not yet clear, but likely involves production of nitric oxide by vascular endothelium.

PHARMACOKINETICS	CONTRAINDICATIONS	DRUG INTERACTIONS	NOTES
PO. Prolonged duration in patients with renal dysfunction. Captopril requires 2–3 doses per day, others one.	Pregnancy. May cause fetal death or injury during second or third trimester. Bilateral renal artery stenosis.	Increased antihypertensive and hypotensive effects with diuretics, sympathetic blockers. Increased serum potassium with potassium-sparing diuretics. Decreased antihypertensive effects with indomethacin.	Often used in conjunction with a thiazide diuretic. Immediate cessation is indicated upon signs of potential angioedema (swelling of face, lips, eyelids or difficulty breathing or swallowing).
PO. Metabolite is 40 times more potent than parent.	Pregnancy.	Phenobarbital reduces level of Losartan and metabolites.	
PO. Once daily.	Serum potassium > 5.5 mEg/L. Creatinine clearance <30 ml/min.	Ketoconazole, itraconazole, other CYP3A4 inhibitors.	
PO/IV/IM. Excreted unchanged and as acetylated metabolites. Rapid acetylators have lower plasma levels than slow acetylators.	Patients with ischemic heart disease.	Potentiates other antihypertensives. Reduces vasoconstriction by sympathomimetic drugs.	Beta-blockers are usually used concomitantly to reduce reflex tachycardia. Diuretics are also used adjunctively to reduce sodium and water retention.
Duration = 24 hours, metabolized by glucuronide conjugation.	" "	Causes profound othostatic hypotension in combination with guanethidine.	Cardiac or pulmonary function impairment may require cessation of drug.
PO			Discontinue if rash develops.
PO. Twice daily dosing		May inhibit Levodopa.	
Continuous infusion IV. Requires pump for home use.	Left ventricle-based congestive heart failure.		
Metabolized to cyanide and cyanmethemoglobin inside red blood cells. Full effect within two minutes and rapid loss of effect when infusion is discontinued.			Dramatic changes in blood pressure occur with small infusion rate changes.
IV. Continuous infusion Halflife = 5 min.			Administer in ICU setting only.

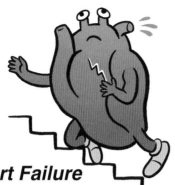

Angina and Heart Failure

• Treatment of Stable Angina

Aspirin reduces the rate of cardiovascular events by 1/3 in patients with stable angina, and should be given to all patients unless they have a clear contraindication. Patients with aspirin allergy should be placed on either ticlopidine or clopidogrel. (Table 4.10). These drugs have not been specifically studied in patients with stable angina, but are effective antiplatelet agents. Neutropenia is much less common in patients treated with clopidogrel than patients treated with ticlopidine.

Beta-blockers (Table 4.2C) reduce the frequency of angina and increase treadmill time in patients with chronic angina. There is less evidence that beta-blockers reduce death in this setting, unless the patient has had a previous infarction.

Calcium channel blockers (Table 4.3) are equally effective as beta-blockers in reducing anginal symptoms in stable patients. Some studies have suggested a higher cardiovascular event rate with short acting dihydropyridines (nifedipine) and these drugs should not be used without a beta blocker. Calcium channel blockers are recommended in patients with vasospastic angina.

Similar to calcium channel blockers and beta blockers, nitrates improve exercise tolerance, and time to onset of angina in patients with exertional stable angina (Table 4.4). Nitrates are contraindicated in

Table 4.3 Antihypertensive/Anti–anginal Agents – Calcium Entry Blockers

DRUG	MECHANISM/ACTIONS	INDICATIONS	UNDESIRABLE EFFECTS
Verapamil (Isopten)	Blocks calcium influx. Dilates peripheral arterioles, reducing afterload. Slows A-V node, prevents reentrant rhythms, protects myocardium during brief ischemia. Has alpha-adrenergic blocking activity.	Reduces frequency of angina and the need for nitrates. Drug of choice for acute paroxysmal supraventricular tachycardia. Slows ventricular response to atrial fibrillation. Hypertension.	Constipation, hypotension, bradycardia, edema, congestive heart failure, A-V node block (rare), GI upset, dizziness.
Diltiazem (Cardizem)	Less pronounced heart rate reduction. Reduces afterload by dilating peripheral arteries. Increases oxygen supply to myocardium by preventing sympathetic-induced coronary artery spasm.	Reduces angina episodes. Increases exercise tolerance in stable angina. Also used as an antihypertensive.	Edema, headache, dizziness, asthenia, nausea, rash.
Nifedipine (Procardia)	More potent peripheral vasodilation. Little depression of nodes. Fails to dilate coronary arteries. Causes reflex increase in heart rate and output.	No longer used as single agent due to toxicity.	Myocardial infarction, peripheral edema, dizziness, nausea, transient hypotension, reflex tachycardia, pulmonary edema.
Nicardipine (Cardene)	Similar to nifedipine	Chronic, stable angina. Hypertension.	" " Fewer myocardial infarctions, more palpitations.
Isradipine (Dynacirc)	Selectively inhibits vascular smooth muscle contraction and S-A node conduction with little effect on heart contractility or A-V node conduction.	Angina, hypertension.	Little tachycardia because of selective actions. Headache, peripheral edema, and flushing.
Felodipine (Plendil)	Peripheral vasodilation, enhanced myocardial contractility and output.	Hypertension.	Peripheral edema, flushing, headache, dizziness.
Amlodipine (Norvasc)	" "	Hypertension, chronic stable angina, vasospastic angina.	Headache, edema, palpitations.
Nisoldipine (Sular)		Hypertension	

Table 4.4 Anti-anginal Agents – Nitrates [a]

DRUG	SUMMARY
Nitroglycerin (Go Nitro)	**Actions:** Dilates large myocardial arteries to increase blood supply to heart. Reduces cardiac preload by reducing venous tone. This allows blood pooling in the periphery. **Indications:** Most commonly used antianginal agent. Useful in treating all forms of angina. May be used immediately before exercise or stress to prevent ischemic episodes. **Undesirable effects:** Hypotension and rebound tachycardia, bradycardia, cerebral ischemia, contact dermatitis may occur with transdermal preparation, aggravation of peripheral edema. **Pharmacokinetics:** Sublingual: peak levels 1–2 min, duration = 30–60 min. IV: Onset by 2 min, duration 3–5 min. Transdermal: peak levels at 30–60 min, duration = 1 day. Topical paste: Onset by 1 hour, duration = 2–12 hours. Once absorbed, liver rapidly metabolizes drug to inactive forms. Tolerance may occur with continuous transdermal adminstration. **Drug Interactions:** Alcohol, antihypertensive agents and vasodilators increase risk of orthostatic hypotension.
Isosorbide dinitrate (Isordil)	Used for prophylaxis of angina. Not for acute attack. Sublingual: onset by 5 min, duration = 1–4 hours. Oral: onset = 30 min, duration = 4–6 hours (up to 8 hours with sustained release formula.)

[a] Beta blockers (Table 4.2C) and calcium entry blockers (Table 4.3) are also used in the treatment of stable angina. Unstable angina is treated with aspirin, heparin (Table 4.9, 4.10)

PHARMACOKINETICS	CONTRAIND.	DRUG INTERACTIONS	NOTES
PO/IV. Well absorbed, 80% metabolized in first pass. 90% protein bound. Metabolites are active. Half-life is 5 hrs but may be up to 20 hrs in patients with cirrhosis.	Patient on IV β-blockers or digitalis. A-V node block, sick sinus syndrome, cardiogenic shock, heart failure, hypotension.	Beta blockers or digitalis: Increases likelihood of bradycardia or A-V blockade. Quinidine or prazosin: Increases hypotension. Digoxin levels are increased. Cimetidine reduces verapamil clearance. Calcium supplements may inhibit actions of verapamil.	Depolarization (leading to contraction) of vascular smooth muscle is dependent on calcium entry. Vasodilation is induced by calcium entry blockers because they inhibit calcium influx.
PO. 50% bioavailability after oral dose. 75% protein bound, half-life = 3 hrs, metabolites are active. Reduce dose in patients with renal dysfunction.	AV node block, sick sinus syndrome, hypotension, pulmonary congestion.	Beta-blockers and digoxin increase A-V conduction time. Diltiazem increases propranolol levels. Cimetidine and drugs metabolized by P-450 increase diltiazem levels.	" "
PO/sublingual. Rapid, complete absorption of sublingual dose. 98%protein bound. Metabolites are inactive, half-life = 3 hrs.	Hypotension.	Betablockers increase risk of severe hypotension, heart failure, and angina. Nifedipine increases effects of oral anticoagulants.	Initial doses may exacerbate angina. Reduce dose in patients with liver dysfunction.
PO/IV. Well absorbed. Reduce dose w/liver-kidney dysfunction.	Severe aortic stenosis.		
PO. Well abosorbed, high first-pass metabolism.			
Slow onset of action (2–5 hours).		Increases digoxin levels.	
PO. Slowest onset, longest halflife.		Increases digoxin and beta blocker effects.	Less acute hypotension due to slow onset.
PO. Once daily.			

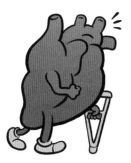

patients taking sildenafil (Viagra). Sildenafil potentiates the hypotensive effects of nitrates and increases the risk of life threatening hypotension.

The drugs discussed above have been tested in combination, and combination therapy is more effective than single drug therapy.

Treatment of Unstable Angina

Rupture of an unstable plaque, and resulting thrombus formation leads to unstable angina. Treatment is targeted toward reducing myocardial demand, improving oxygen delivery, reducing coronary spasm, and halting thrombus formation. Heparin has been the primary anticoagulant. Recent trials have revealed the importance of antiplatelet therapy.

Oxygen therapy improves oxygen delivery in the subset of patients who are hypoxemic from CHF or underlying lung disease. Morphine reduces the pain and anxiety that can worsen symptoms in many patients. Treating these symptoms can reduce the myocardial demand, reducing the total amount of ischemia.

Medications that directly decrease cardiac workload are effective in unstable angina. Beta blockers reduce ischemic burden by decreasing heart rate and blood pressure (Table 4.2C). This class of medications may reduce further myocardial infarctions by 10–20%. Nitrates are extremely effective in reducing symptoms by decreasing

blood pressure and inducing coronary vasodilation (Table 4.4). Although nitrates clearly reduce symptoms, there is no convincing evidence that they reduce mortality or the rate of myocardial infarctions. Calcium channel blockers must be considered as two classes: dihydropyridines (i.e. nifedipine) and non-dihydropyridines (i.e. diltiazem, Table 4.3). It is important to note that nifedipine can be hazardous in this setting, leading to a higher rate of myocardial infarction or recurrent angina if given without a beta blocker. Non-dihydropyridine calcium channel blockers (i.e. diltiazem) can be safely used and may reduce the rate of death or recurrent myocardial infarction. This class of medicines is an excellent choice in patients with absolute contraindications to beta blockers.

Heparin has proven effective in the setting of unstable angina in many studies, reducing the rate of myocardial infarction or death by up to 35% when used in addition to aspirin (Table 4.9). Weight based protocols have become more popular in the wake of studies that have demonstrated their superiority over non weight based treatment. More recently, low molecular weight heparin (i.e. enoxaparin) has proven more effective than unfractionated heparin in the setting of unstable angina. All low-molecular weight heparins are not equal. Other LMWH's have not proven superiority over heparin in the setting of unstable angina.

Antiplatelet therapy has also been studied carefully. Aspirin therapy has reduced the rate of recurrent ischemia, infarctions and death by more than 50%.

Two newer antiplatelets, derivatives of thienopyridines, have recently been added (Table 4.10). Ticlopidine (Ticlid) has been most extensively studied in the field of ischemic cerebrovascular events, and reduced the rate of vascular events compared to aspirin. It does carry an increased risk of neutropenia and rarely can cause thrombotic thrombocytopenic purpura. Clopidogrel (Plavix) has been compared to aspirin and was more effective in preventing recurrent

Table 4.5A Drugs used for stable congestive heart failure/cardiomyopathy

DRUG	MECH/ACTIONS	INDICATIONS	UNDESIRABLE EFFECTS
Beta blockers (Tables 2.4 & 4.2C)	Agents that preferentially block β1 adrenergic receptors decrease heart rate and output and reduce renin release.	Metaprolol is indicated for congestive heart failure. Metaprolol, atenolol, propranolol and timolol are indicated for post-myocardial infarction patients. Many are indicated for hypertension.	CNS sedation and depression. Not indicated for acute or severe heart failure.
ACE inhibitors (Table 4.2D)	Reduces peripheral arterial resistance in hypertensive patients, by inhibiting angiotensin converting enzyme (ACE).	Chronic congestive heart failure. Mild to moderate hypertension.	See Table 4.2D
Aldosterone inhibitors (e.g. spironolactone, eplerenone)	Aldosterone antagonist is a diuretic that reduces blood volume (Table 4.2A).	Congestive heart failure, cirrhosis, nephrotic syndrome.	Hyperkalemia, sodium or water depletion, endocrine imbalances.

ischemic events in patients with vascular disease. Although neither thienopyridine has been studied specifically in unstable angina, they are accepted substitutes for those patients that cannot take aspirin.

Adjunctive Treatment of Myocardial Infarction

Thrombolytic therapy reduces the relative risk of death by 20% if given within the first 12 hours of an acute infarction. There are several types of thrombolytic agents available (Table 4.10). Accelerated dose alteplase reduced mortality further than streptokinase in a very large study (GUSTO). Since then, other tissue plasminogen activators have been developed that are easier to dose. These drugs should only be used in the setting of ST elevation. Thrombolysis is not effective when the patient's ECG shows only ST depression or no diagnostic changes. In fact, there is evidence that thrombolysis is dangerous in non-ST elevation ischemic syndromes.

Drugs that inhibit clot formation and extension include:

1. Heparin or low molecular weight heparin
2. IIb/IIIa inhibitors (prevent platelets from sticking), eg tirofiban, eptifibatide and abciximab
3. Aspirin

Aspirin by itself reduces the risk of death from an infarction by 23%. It has an additive effect when used in combination with a thrombolytic medication. Aspirin should always be used in the setting of an infarction unless the patient has evidence of an active gastrointestinal bleed, or a true allergy to aspirin. In the setting of an allergy, clopidogrel (Plavix) can be substituted for aspirin.

Beta blockers (Table 4.2C) reduce chest pain, myocardial wall stress and infarct size in the setting of an infarct.

Over 50,000 patients have been enrolled in studies designed to evaluate the effects of beta blockers during or after an infarction. The evidence overwhelmingly suggests that beta blockers reduce death after myocardial infarction, and these drugs should be given in all patients with acute myocardial infarction who do not have clear contraindications such as pulmonary edema, hypotension, bradycardia, advanced heart block or asthma.

Angiotensin inhibitors (Table 4.2D) have been convincingly shown to dramatically decrease death rates in patients with reduced left ventricular dysfunction after an infarction. These drugs also reduce death in all patients after myocardial infarction but the relative risk reduction of death is much less powerful. ACE inhibitors also reduce the rate of progression to heart failure. ACE inhibitors should be given in all patients presenting with an acute myocardial infarction, unless they have contraindications such as renal failure, bilateral renal insufficiency, hypotension, or angioedema due to previous ACE inhibitor use.

Nitrate therapy has not consistently reduced death or recurrent infarction in these patients (Table 4.4). This class of medications does reduce ischemic chest pain and should be used for symptomatic patients.

Calcium-channel blockers do not reduce mortality during or after acute myocardial infarction. Diltiazem may reduce the rate of recurrent infarction after a non Q wave infarct, but any advantage over aspirin and beta blockers is not known. There may be an adverse effect of short acting dihydropyridines (nifedipine) and these drugs should be avoided in this setting.

Antiarrhythmic drugs have been studied in the setting of acute infarctions. Class I and Class III drugs have increased the rate of death compared to placebo when used to suppress ventricular ectopy after myocardial infarctions, especially in patients with reduced left ventricular function.

PHARMACOKINETICS	CONTRAINDICATIONS	DRUG INTERACTIONS	NOTES
See Tables 2.4 & 4.2C	Sinus bradycardia, severe heart failure. Agents with b2 blocking activity contraindicated in asthma or COPD patients.	See Tables 2.4 & 4.2C.	
See Table 4.2D.	See Table 4.2D.	See Table 4.2D.	
PO. Metabolized extensively in liver to active metabolite. Metabolite is 98% protein bound, therefore the halflife is 1–1.5 days.	Anuria, renal insufficiency, hyperkalemia, diabetes.	Increases risk of digoxin toxicity and decreases vasopressor action of norepinephrine.	The metabolite, canrenone, is primarily responsible for drug actions.

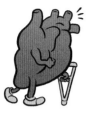

Heart Failure Drugs

• Acute Pulmonary Edema

Acute pulmonary edema usually accompanies left heart failure. Successful treatment of pulmonary edema reduces the risk of secondary right heart failure. Early interventions in patients with pulmonary edema include (1) sitting the patient upright to decrease venous return and ease breathing and (2) administering humidified oxygen to increase PaO_2.

Drug therapy consists of (1) furosemide or bumetanide, potent diuretics which reduce vascular volume, leading to a shift of fluid from the lungs into the vasculature; and (2) morphine, a venodilator which decreases preload and reduces anxiety through its action on opiate receptors in the brain (Tables 4.3A & 3.6A). Nitrates and/or bronchodilators may be added to reduce ischemic damage and improve ventilation, respectively (Tables 4.4 & 5.1).

• Management of Shock

Shock is a potentially fatal condition in which tissues are poorly perfused and, consequently, become ischemic.

Table 4.5B Other Heart Failure Drugs

DRUG	MECHANISM/ACTIONS	INDICATIONS	UNDESIRABLE EFFECTS
Cardiac glycosides			
Digoxin (Lanoxin)	Inhibits Na$^+$/K$^+$-ATPase (sodium pump) and ↑ inward current of Ca^{++}. Contraction enhanced by ↑ intracellular Ca^{++}. ↑ cardiac output and ↓ heart size, venous return, and blood volume. Causes diuresis by ↑ renal perfusion. Slows ventricular rate in atrial fibrillation or flutter by ↑ sensitivity of AV nodes to vagal inhibition. ↑ peripheral vascular resistance.	Heart failure, atrial fibrillation, atrial flutter, paroxysmal tachycardia. Also indicated for hypoventilation, cardiogenic shock and thyrotoxic shock. Often a loading dose is administered first to achieve therapeutic concentrations more rapidly.	Digitalis intoxication (See text), bradycardia, AV or SA node block, arrhythmias. Also anorexia, nausea, vomiting, diarrhea, headache, fatigue, malaise, visual disturbances, and gynecomastia. Increased peripheral resistance may increase the heart's workload, worsening ischemic damage.
Bipyridine derivatives			
Milrinone (Primacor)	Inhibits phosphodiesterase (the enzyme that breaks down cAMP). cAMP increases calcium uptake. Increases contractility, stroke volume, ejection fraction, and sinus rate. Decreases peripheral resistance.	Added to digoxin therapy when heart failure persists despite digoxin. Has not been shown to be effective in heart failure that lasts >48 hrs.	Ventricular arrhythmias. Requires constant ECG monitoring.
Other agents			
Dobutamine (Dobutrex)	Beta$_1$ receptor-preferring adrenergic agonist. At moderate dose, increases contractility without increasing heart rate or blood pressure. Minimal effect on blood vessels.	To increase cardiac output in chronic heart failure. May be used with afterload reducing agents. Also used for treatment of shock.	Tachycardia, hypotension, nausea, headache, palpitations, anginal symptoms, dyspnea, ventricular arrhythmias.
Terazosin (Hytrin)	" "	Heart failure.	Light headedness, fatigue, headache, GI distress, nasal congestion, tachycardia, edema.
Vasodilators	Described in detail in Table 4.2D		
Nesiritide (Natrecor)	Brain Natriuretic Peptide analog.	Heart failure.	Hypotension
Ivabradine (Corlanor)	Blocks the hyperpolarization-activated cyclic nucleotide-gated channel.	Chronic heart failure in patients who are on maximum dose of beta blockers	Bradycardia, hypertension, atrial fibrillation, visual brightness.

Treatment consists of maintaining oxygenation, supporting blood pressure and treating the metabolic acidosis if it is severe. The type of shock must be diagnosed so that the underlying problem can be treated.

Vasopressors constrict blood vessels and improve cardiac function by stimulating adrenergic receptors (Table 2.1). They are employed when intravenous fluids alone fail to increase central venous pressure. Peripheral vasoconstriction shunts blood to the heart and lungs. It may seem odd that vasoconstrictors are used to treat a condition marked by poor tissue perfusion. Indeed, improvement in central venous pressure is frequently at the expense of ischemic damage to peripheral tissues.

Low-dose dopamine is the preferred agent for treating shock. At "renal doses", dopamine dilates renal vessels (dopamine receptor-mediated) while constricting vessels in other tissues. Norepinephrine and high-dose dopamine constrict all vessels including those of the kidney and brain. In addition, both of these agents improve cardiac function by stimulating β_1 adrenergic receptors. Dopamine is more potent than norepinephrine in this regard.

Dobutamine and isoproterenol are also used in cardiogenic shock because they improve myocardial contractility. These agents are contraindicated when shock is due to hypovolemia rather than cardiac insufficiency, because they have no direct vasoconstrictor effects (weak α_1 agonists). Dobutamine must be used with caution in patients with systolic blood pressure less than 100 because it can worsen hypotension.

PHARMACOKINETICS	CONTRAINDICATIONS	DRUG INTERACTIONS	NOTES
PO/IV. 36 hr half-life, 75% absorbed in GI tract, slow distribution due to large apparent volume of distribution (reduced in elderly), excreted unchanged in urine (but does adjustment unnecessary w/renal dysfunction), 25% protein bound.	Ventricular fibrillation, severe bradycardia, allergic reaction to cardiac glycosides.	Increased risk of toxicity with drugs that alter serum electrolytes (potassium- depleting diuretics, corticosteroids, thiazide and loop diuretics, amphotericin B, quinidine, amiodarone). Blockers of β adrenergic receptors, calcium channels, or acetylcholinesterase increase risk of complete AV block. Drugs which alter GI absorption may alter bioavailability.	ECG effects: T wave diminished in amplitude or inverted, P-R interval prolonged, Q-T interval shortened. Tests for serum digoxin levels may be altered by electrolyte imbalance, renal impairment, age, thyroid disease, other drugs, or substances in the body which imitate dioxin in radioimmunoassay.
IV. Well absorbed, short half-life (1.5 hrs).			If cellular supplies of cAMP are depleted, milrinone will not be effective. Capable of increasing myocardial contraction even in the presence of β-adrenergic antagonists.
IV. 2.4 min half-life. Continuous infusion is necessary to maintain therapeutic effect.	Hypersensitivity to dobutamine. Idiopathic hypertrophic subaortic stenosis.	None identified.	Because of short half-life, can only be used for short-term therapy.
PO. All patients MUST start with 1 mg dose before bed, then increase dose slowly if hypotension is not a problem.		" "	
IV. Short half-life	Cardiogenic shock.		
PO. Food delays absorption and increases plasma exposure.	Acute decompensating heart failure. BP < 90/50.	Concomitant use of strong CYP3A4 inhibitors increases ivabradine levels.	Goal is to reduce the risk of hospitalization

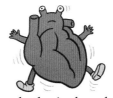

Arrhythmias

The following tables present arrhythmias based on the anatomical site of the underlying abnormality – atrial, ventricular or supraventricular

(A-V junction) accessory pathway. Arrhythmias occur because one or more regions of the heart are 1) beating too slowly (sinus bradycardia); 2) beating too fast (sinus or ventricular tachycardia, atrial or ventricular premature depolarization, atrial flutter); 3) beating automatically without regard for impulses originating from the SA node (multifocal atrial tachycardia, atrial fibrillation, ventricular fibrillation), or 4) allowing impulses to travel along an accessory pathway to areas of the heart which should not be depolarized at that particular moment (A-V reentry, Wolff-Parkinson-White syndrome).

Table 4.6A Arrhythmias

CLASSIFICATION/PATHOLOGY		ECG FINDINGS
Arrhythmias Originating in the Atrium		
Sinus Bradycardia: Increased parasympathetic (vagal) tone causes heart to beat at <60 beats per minute. Depolarization originates from sinoatrial node (hence the name sinus).	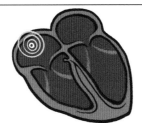	Slow, but regular rate on rhythm strip.
Sinus Tachycardia: Increased sympathetic tone causes heart to race (100–160 beats per minute). Depolarization originates from sinoatrial node.	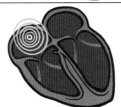	Rapid, but regular rate on rhythm strip.
Multifocal Atrial Tachycardia. Depolarization originates from several atrial foci at irregular intervals. Rate is rapid (100–200 beats per minute) and irregular.	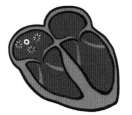	P waves are present, but are morphologically different from one another. P-R interval varies.
Premature Atrial Depolarization (PAT): Heart beats prematurely because a focus of atrial cells fires spontaneously before the SA node is ready to fire.	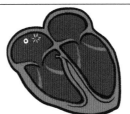	Interruption of regular rhythm by an early P wave. P wave may be followed by a norma QRS if the SA node and ventricle have had time to repolarize.
Atrial Flutter: Atrial impulse reenters and depolarizes atrium. Generates 250–350 impulses per minute. The ventricle responds to every 2nd or 3rd impulse. Both atrial and ventricular rhythm are regular.	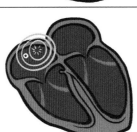	Series of 2–4 closely spaced P waves followed by a normal QRS complex. 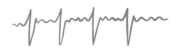

Table 4.6B Arrhythmias (cont.)

CLASSIFICATION/PATHOLOGY   **ECG FINDINGS**

Arrhythmias Originating in the Atrium (cont.)

Atrial Fibrillation:
Multiple ectopic foci of atrial cells generate 350–450 impulses per minute. The ventricle responds to an occasional impulse. Both atrial and ventricular rhythm are irregular.

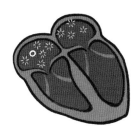

P waves can not be discerned. Baseline is irregular with unevenly-spaced QRS complexes.

Arrhythmias Involving the A-V Junction

A-V Reentry: A-V node is split into a pathway which conducts toward the ventricle and a pathway which conducts the impulse BACK to the atrium. Reentry of the impulse into the atrium causes the atrium and ventricle to contract simultaneously.

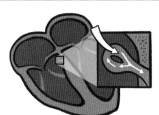

Generally normal QRS complexes following normal P waves. The inverted P wave (retrograde atrial contraction) is buried in the QRS. Rate is 150–250/minute.

Wolff-Parkinson-White:
A strip of conducting tissue (other than the A-V node) connects the atrium and ventricle. Impulses reaching the ventricle via the A-V node circle back to the atrium via the accessory pathway. Alternatively, the circuit may be reversed.

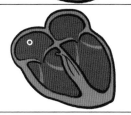

Each P wave is followed rapidly by a QRS. A "delta wave" leads into the QRS. Rate can exceed 300 beats/minute.

Arrhythmias Originating in the Ventricle

Ventricular Premature Depolarization:
Spontaneous depolarization of ectopic focus in the ventricle. Considered benign if fewer than six per minute.

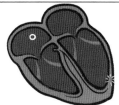

Wide, tall QRS complexes which are not associated with a P wave. A prominent T wave often points in the opposite direction as the QRS complex.

Ventricular Tachycardia: Usually secondary to reentry circuit. Both A-V reentry and Wolff-Parkinson-White may progress to ventricular tachycardia.

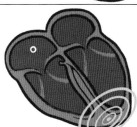

Wide QRS complexes with abnormal S-T segment and T wave deflections (opposite in direction to QRS). AV dissociation and right bundle branch block are often associated.

Ventricular Fibrillation:
Erratic discharge from many ectopic foci in the ventricle. Rate is 350–450 beats/min. Rhythm is irregular.

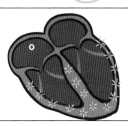

Completely erratic. Cannot distinguish normal waves or complexes.

Antiarrhythmic Agents

The sinoatrial node paces the heart by spontaneously depolarizing and stimulating the conducting nerves of the atrium. The impulse rapidly spreads through the atrium, causing myocardial cells of the atrium to contract in unison. The impulse reaches the atrioventricular (A-V) node, which in turn transmits the conduction signal to the His-Purkinje conduction pathway. The His-Purkinje system carries the impulse to ventricular myocardial cells, causing a powerful contraction that propels blood throughout the body.

Interruption of this magnificent system, by the mechanisms described in Table 4.6, jeopardizes tissue oxygenation and may lead to death. Antiarrhythmic drugs influence cardiac conduction properties (usually by modifying ion conductance) and may revert an abnormal rhythm to sinus rhythm.

An understanding of the mechanism by which action potentials are propagated through conducting cells facilitates learning about the mechanism of antiarrythmic action (Fig. 4.2).

Antiarrhythmic drugs have been divided into four classes to facilitate comparison and discussion. Since the time the drugs were classified, however, it has become clear that drugs within each class may differ significantly and cannot be substituted for one another. The original classification scheme (bold-face print) and other generalizations include:

Table 4.7A Antiarrhythmic Drugs

DRUG	MECHANISM/ACTION	INDICATIONS	UNDESIRABLE EFFECTS
Class I			
Quinidine	Depresses automaticity of ectopic foci. Slows conduction velocity in atria & His-Purkinje cells. Prolongs refractory period throughout heart (except nodes) and accessory pathways. Has anticholinergic effects which may actually enhance A-V conduction in patients with rapid atrial depolarization.	Multifocal atrial tachycardia, premature atrial depolarization, premature ventricular depolarization, atrial fibrillation (these result from increased automaticity of ectopic foci), and ventricular tachycardia.	Torsades de pointes (recurrent, temporary arrhythmia), increases ventricle response to atrial tachyarrhythmia, nausea, vomiting, diarrhea, hypersensitivity, cinchonism, thrombocytopenic purpura.
Procainamide (e.g., Pronestyl)	" "	Premature atrial depolarization, atrial fibrillation, Wolff-Parkinson-White, ventricular tachycardia, atrial flutter, premature ventricular depolarization.	Fewer GI effects and weaker anticholinergic effects than quinidine, but similar cardiac toxicity. Lupus-like syndrome and other hypersensitivity reactions.
Disopyramide (e.g., Norpace)	" "	Premature atrial depolarization, Atrial fibrillation, Ventricular tachycardia	Potent anticholinergic effects. Otherwise similar to quinidine.
Lidocaine (e.g., Xylocaine)	Depresses automaticity of ectopic foci, increases conduction velocity of A-V node and His-Purkinje.	Wolff-Parkinson-White, Ventricular tachycardia, Premature vent. depolarization, Ventricular fibrillation.	CNS: paresthesias, drowsiness, confusion, restlessness (at low doses). At high doses, seizures or disorientation. Cardiac depression (if given by rapid IV), arrhythmias.
Mexiletine (Mexitil)	Decreases automaticity of AV node and ectopic foci. Prolongs refractory period of His-Purkinje, ventricle, and accessory pathway.	Premature vent. depolarization, Ventricular tachycardia (life-threatening ventricular arrhythmias).	May worsen arrhythmias, hepatotoxicity, rarely convulsions
Flecainide (Tambocor)	Reduces 1) automaticity of SA node & ectopic foci, 2) conduction velocity throughout. Prolongs refractory period in His-Purkinje, ventricle, and accessory pathways.	Chronic therapy for atrial fibrillation.	May worsen arrhythmias. Rarely induces A-V block in patients with A-V conduction delay.
Propafenone (Rhythmol)	Slows conduction throughout, prolongs atrial and ventricular refractory period, has weak β adrenergic and calcium-entry blocking effects.	Chronic or acute therapy for atrial fibrillation.	Nausea, dizziness, constipation, altered taste sensation. May worsen heart failure or arrhythmias.

- **Class I drugs are Na+ channel blockers.** Class Ia drugs have little effect on SA node automaticity, while most other antiarrhythmics reduce SA node automaticity. Class Ia drugs slow conduction velocity and tend to be more effective than other classes in prolonging the refractory period. No clear generalizations can be made of Class Ib agents. Class Ic drugs slow conduction velocity most effectively.
- **Class II drugs antagonize adrenergic receptors.**
- **Class III agents tend to prolong repolarization.**
- **Class IV agents block slow inward (calcium driven) current.**
- Automaticity is suppressed in ectopic foci by every antiarrhythmic except bretylium.

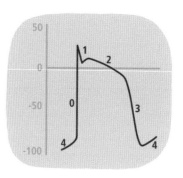

Figure 4.2 Example of action potential in cardiac conducting cells. Phase 0: Voltage-dependent Na^+ channel opens and rapid sodium influx depolarizes cell. Phase 1: Rapid phase of repolarization caused by inactivation of Na^+ influx and the activation of a transient outward K^+ current. Phase 2: Plateau phase, characterized by low membrane conductance and the activation of a slow inward Ca^{++} current. Phase 3. Repolarization to resting potential results from outward K^+ current. Phase 4. Outward K^+ current is deactivated and an inward $Na+$ current reduces transmembrane potential.

ECG CHANGES	PHARMACOKINETICS	DRUG INTERACTIONS	NOTES
Prolongs QRS and QT intervals.	PO best/IM painful/IV causes hypotension. 90% protein bound. Primarily metabolized in liver, excreted by kidney. Adjust dose by monitoring plasma level. Extended duration formula allows BID dosing.	Phenobarbital and phenytoin increase metabolism of quinidine. Quinidine increases plasma levels of digoxin, enhances vasodilator-induced hypotension and potentiates warfarin.	
" "	PO/IM/IV. Low protein binding, otherwise like quinidine. The metabolite, N-acetylprocainamide (NAPA) is active and toxic. NAPA levels should be monitored.	No interaction with digoxin or warfarin.	
" "	PO only. 50% metabolized by liver, 50% excreted unchanged. Must follow serum levels.	No interaction with digoxin.	
May shorten QT interval.	IV, rarely IM. Rapidly metabolized by liver (2 metabolites are active), excreted by kidney.	Serum level increased by drugs which reduce blood flow to liver (β blockers) and by cimetidine.	
ECG changes not detectable.	PO. Maintain dose <1.2 g/day to reduce risk of CNS toxicity. Extensive metabolism in liver.	P450-inducing drugs (rifampin, phenytoin) reduce half-life of mexiletine.	
Prolongs PR, QRS and QT.	PO/IV. GI absorption varies widely between patients. 10% of the population metabolizes the drug slowly (4 times slower than remaining 90% of population.)	Effects additive with other drugs which affect heart conduction. Cimetidine increases half-life of encainide.	Class Ic agents may cause mortality in patients with structural heart disease. Avoid in patients with non-life-threatening ventricular arrhythmias.
" "	PO. 10% of the population, metabolizes the drug slowly, prolonging the half-life substantially. Titrate doses carefully.	Propafenone increases plasma levels of propranolol, digoxin and warfarin. Cimetidine increases propafenone levels.	" "

Table 4.7B Antiarrhythmic Drugs (cont.)

DRUG	MECHANISM/ACTIONS	INDICATIONS	UNDESIRABLE EFFECTS
Class II			
Propranolol (Inderal)	β adrenergic receptor antagonist. ↓ heart rate, contractility and automaticity. Prolongs A-V conduction time and refractoriness.	Sinus tachycardia, atrial flutter, atrial fibrillation, A-V reentry, Wolff-Parkinson-White	Heart failure, depressed A-V conduction, bronchospasm, hypotension.
Esmolol (Kerlone)	β1 adrenergic receptor-preferring antagonist. Similar to propranolol in action.	" "	Less likely to cause bronchospasm than propranolol. Otherwise similar.
Class III			
Amiodarone	Reduces potassium efflux. Reduces automaticity of SA node and ectopic foci, reduces conduction velocity and increases refractoriness.	Effective inhibitor of ventricular fibrillation, ventricular tachycardia, Wolff-Parkinson-White, atrial fibrillation.	Corneal deposits (reversible), hypo- or hyper- thyroidism (T4- like structure), photosensitivity, pulmonary fibrosis, bradycardia (rarely severe).
Sotalol (Betapace)	Beta adrenergic blocker that slows refractory period of Purkinje fibers & heart muscle.	Ventricular tachycardia.	Arrhythmias.
Dofetilide (Tikosyn)	Blocks the rapid component of the delayed rectifier outward potassium current.	Atrial fibrillation or atrial flutter	Tachycardia, irregular heartbeat, rash, diarrhea, dizziness, vomiting, sweating, loss of appetite, thirst.
Ibutilide (Corvert)	Prolongs the action potential duration and increases both atrial and ventricular refractoriness.	Atrial fibrillation or atrial flutter	Tachycardia, premature ventricular contractions, A-V block, bundle branch block, hypotension, prolonged QT interval.
Class IV			
Verapamil	Reduces 1) Ca^{++} entry into myocardial cells, 2) SA node and ectopic foci automaticity, 3) conduction and increases refractory period of AV node.	Multifocal atrial tachycardia, atrial flutter	Sinus bradycardia, AV block, hypotension, GI upset, constipation. If infused rapidly into elderly patients, may cause left ventricular failure.
Unclassified			
Digoxin (Lanoxin)	Only drug which increases automaticity of ectopic pacemakers. Slows conduction velocity throughout. Complex actions on refractory period. Increases parasympathetic tone.	Atrial fibrillation, atrial flutter, paroxysmal atrial tachycardia.	See Table 4.2A. digitalis intoxication, arrhythmias, vomiting, headache, visual distrurbances. Complete heart block and accelerated junctional rhythm.
Adenosine (Adenocard)	Decreases conduction velocity, prolongs refractory period and decreases automaticity in A-V node.	Paroxysmal supraventricular tachyarrhythmias.	Dyspnea, flushing, chest pain, arrhythmias.

ECG CHANGES	PHARMACOKINETICS	DRUG INTERACTIONS	NOTES
Slow heart rate. Prolong PR and QT interval.	PO/IV. 90% protein bound, Metabolized by liver, excreted by kidney.	Possibly fatal A-V node block when combined with digitalis.	
" "	IV. Metabolized by erythrocyte esterase. Metabolite excreted renally. Serum levels unaffected by liver or kidney failure.	No significant interactions with digoxin.	
Prolong PR, QRS and QT.	PO/IV. Maximal response may take weeks. Serum levels correspond poorly w/efficacy.	Increases serum levels of digoxin, warfarin, flecainide.	
	PO. Reduce dose with renal dysfunction.	Increased risk of arrhythmias with other antiarrhythmics.	
Prolongs corrected QT interval	PO. Steady state levels are achieved in 2-3 days.	Diuretics, verapamil, trimethoprim, cimetidine, ketoconazole, megastrol	Contraindicated if QTc or QT > 440 msec
Prolongs corrected QT interval	PO. Metabolized in liver. Halflife 2-12 hours.	Cisapride, dronedarone, thioridazine, pimozide.	Caution advised if QT interval is prolonged.
Slow heart rate, prolong PR interval.	PO/IV. Good GI absorption, but 80% is metabolized in first pass through liver. Half-life increases up to fourfold in cirrhotic patients. Metabolites are active.	Increases serum digoxin levels. Enhances A-V node suppression of digoxin or propranolol - may progress to A-V block.	Contraindicated in Wolff-Parkinson-White (may induce potentially fatal arrhythmia.)
Slows rate, prolongs PR interval, shortens QT interval, diminishes amplitude of T wave.	PO/IV. 36 hour half-life excreted unchanged in urine, 25% protein bound.	See Table 4.2A.	
Increases heart rate and prolongs PR interval.	IV. Rapidly (<30 seconds) deaminated in serum to active agent, inosine.	Theophylline and other methylxanthines antagonize adenosine.	

Lipid-lowering Agents

Lipoproteins are serum transport vehicles for lipids and triglycerides. There are six classes of lipoproteins, which differ with respect to lipid and protein content, transport, function and mechanism of lipid delivery. They are named according to their size and density. Chylomicrons and chylomicron remnants carry lipids that are absorbed through the intestine (exogenous pathway). The other four lipoproteins form the endogenous transport pathway that delivers cholesterol and triglycerides secreted by the liver. The four lipoproteins of the endogenous pathway are very low density lipoprotein (VLDL), intermediate density lipoprotein (IDL), low density lipoprotein (LDL) and high density lipoprotein (HDL).

Elevated lipoprotein concentration contributes to the formation of atherosclerotic plaques and in some cases pancreatitis. Treatment strategies focus first on diet and correction of underlying metabolic diseases. Diets that are low in cholesterol and saturated animal fats reduce lipoprotein levels. In addition, overweight patients should reduce their total caloric intake. Exercise increases serum concentrations of HDL, which is associated with reduced risk of coronary artery disease. Secondary hyperlipidemia frequently subsides upon treatment of the underlying metabolic disease or cessation of aggravating factors.

Drug therapy is generally reserved for patients who fail to respond to diet or other measures described above. Lipid-lowering agents are described in Table 4.8. Strategies for reducing lipid levels included: 1) reducing endogenous cholesterol synthesis, 2) enhancing cholesterol excretion, 3) inhibiting synthesis of lipoproteins, 4) enhancing degradation of lipoproteins. Drugs that work by different mechanisms are sometimes combined to achieve a greater reduction in lipoproteins than possible by monodrug therapy.

All drugs are administered orally. Side effects include GI distress and rash. Most agents potentiate oral anticoagulants. Statins may result in liver and muscle injury.

Anticoagulants, Antiplatelet Agents, and Thrombolytics

Anticoagulants inhibit blood coagulation, **antiplatelet agents** prevent platelet aggregation, and **thrombolytic agents** degrade clots that have already formed.

Table 4.8 Drugs Used to Treat Lipid Disorders

DRUG	MECHANISM/ACTIONS	INDICATIONS	LIPID PROFILE EFFECTS
Cholestyramine (Questran) **Colestipol** (Colestid) **Colesevelam** (Welchol)	Forms insoluble complex with bile salts, excreted in feces. Body compensates by increasing LDL receptors and oxidizing cholesterol.	LDL > 190 mg/dl (160 with 2 risk factors) provided that 6 month trial of low lipid diet has failed.	↓ Cholesterol, LDL ↑ Triglycerides, VLDL, HDL
Lovastatin (Mevacor) **Pravastatin** (Pravachol) **Simvastatin** (Zocor) **Fluvastatin** (Lescol) **Atorvastatin** (Lipitor) **Rosuvastatin** (Crestor)	Inhibit HMG-CoA reductase in liver. This enzyme catalyzes the rate-limiting step in cholesterol synthesis.	" "	↓ Cholesterol, LDL, VLDL, triglyc. ↑ HDL
Pitavastatin (Livalo)			
Gemfibrozil (Lopid)	Inhibits VLDL synthesis, increases lipoprotein lipase activity.	" "	↓ Cholest., triglyc., VLDL, IDL ↓ or ↑ LDL ↑ HDL
Fenofibrate (Tricor)	Unknown	Hypertriglyceridemia	↓ Cholesterol, Triglycerides ↑ LDL, HDL
Ezetimibe (Zetia)	Inhibits cholesterol GI absorption	Hypercholesterolemia	↓ LDL, ↑ HDL, ↓ triglyc.
Evolocumab (Repatha) **Alirocumab** (Praluent)	Antibody that blocks PCSK9, which reduces LDLR	Familial Hypercholesterolemia	Lowers LDL-C levels
Lomitapide (Juxtapid)	Inhibits microsomal triglyceride transfer protein (MTP)	Familial Hypercholesterolemia	GI disorders, chest pain

All drugs are administered orally. Side effects include GI distress and rash. Most agents potentiate oral anticoagulants.

Blood coagulation occurs as a "cascade" of proteolytic factors are activated. Each factor is proteolyzed into an active protease. The newly-formed protease in turn proteolyzes fibrin, which forms an insoluble network that entangles blood cells and platelets.

Several clotting factors require vitamin K for activation. Inhibition of vitamin K is therefore a pharmacologic strategy for preventing coagulation (Table 4.9). The other clinically useful anticoagulation strategy involves inactivating coagulation Factor III, which prevents activation of the coagulation cascade from the extrinsic pathway (Table 4.9).

Thromboxane and some prostaglandins serve as mediators of platelet aggregation. Antithrombotic agents inhibit prostaglandin and thromboxane synthesis (Table 4.10). Alternatively, prostaglandins that *inhibit* platelet aggregation may be used to prevent thrombosis. Once a thrombus has formed, the only clinically-useful pharmacologic strategy involves degrading fibrin with thrombolytic agents (Table 4.10).

Table 4.9 Anticoagulants (see also Table 4.10)

	HEPARIN	WARFARIN (COUMADIN)
Mechanism/Action:	Binds to antithrombin III. This complex then binds to and inhibits activated clotting factors (factor Xa). Larger amounts inactivate thrombin and clotting factors to prevent conversion of fibrinogen to fibrin.	Antagonize vitamin K. Interfere with the synthesis of vitamin K-dependent clotting factors (II, VII, IX, X).
Indications:	Preventing postoperative deep vein thrombosis and pulmonary embolism. Maintaining extracorporeal circulation during open heart surgery and renal hemodialysis. Achieving immediate anticoagulation.	Deep venous thrombosis, ischemic heart disease (selected patients), rheumatic heart disease, pulmonary embolism. Lifelong use in patients with artificial heart valves.
Undesirable Effects:	Bleeding, hemorrhage, thrombocytopenia, hematoma or necrosis at injection site.	Bleeding, necrosis, GI upset.
Pharmacokinetics:	SubQ/IV. Only anticoagulant commonly used parenterally. Dose-dependent kinetics. Metabolized in liver to inactive products.	PO. Well absorbed rapidly, 99% plasma protein bound, half-life = 37 hrs, metabolized by liver.
Drug Interactions:	Risk of bleeding or hemorrhage is increased with concomitant administration of aspirin, ibuprofen, anticoagulants/thrombolytics, dextran, phenylbutazone, indomethacin, dipyridamole, several penicillins and cephalosporins, valproic acid, plicamycin, methimazole, propylthiouracil, probenecid, hydroxychloroquine, chloroquine. Decreased anticoagulation effect with digitalis, tetracyclines, antihistamines, nicotine.	Urokinase and streptokinase increase risk of bleeding. Anticoagulation effects are increased by aspirin, phenylbutazone, oxyphenbutazone, disulfiram, cimetidine, sulfinpyrazone, metronidazole, trimethoprim-sulfamethoxazole, dextrothyroxine, anabolic steroids, heparin, and many others. Anticoagulation effects are decreased by drugs which induce P-450 enzymes, rifampin, cholestryramine, high dose vitamin C or K.
Notes:	Because of hemorrhage risk, check hematocrit and test for blood in stool. Administer with caution to menstruating women, or patients with subacute bacterial endocarditis, severe hypotension, liver disease, or blood dyscrasias. *Protamine sulfate inactivates heparin* and can be used as an antagonist if severe bleeding occurs.	Prothrombin time should be monitored carefully in patients taking warfarin. However, ecchymoses, hematuria, uterine and intestinal bleeding, and other signs of hemorrhage may occur even when prothrombin time is within normal range.
Related drugs:	Low molecular weight heparins [**dalteparin** (Fragmin), **tinzaparin** (Innohep)] and **heparinoids** [**enoxaparin** (Lovenox)] are used for prophylaxis or treatment of deep venous thrombosis and pulmonary emboli. Aldeparin and Enoxaparin also reduce risk of ischemia in unstable angina or non-Q-wave myocardial infarction. These do not alter PT or PTT. Increase risk of spinal/epidural hematoma following lumbar puncture. Lepirudin (Refludan), bivalirudin (Angiomax), and Argatroban are direct thrombin inhibitors.	

Table 4.10 Antiplatelet and Thrombolytic Agents and Direct Thrombin Inhibitors (see also Table 4.9)

DRUG	MECHANISM/ACTIONS	INDICATIONS	UNDESIRABLE EFFECTS
Ticagrelor (Brilinta) **Prasugrel** (Effient)	Binds to the $P2Y_{12}$ class of adenosine diphosphate (ADP) receptors on platelets.	Reduce thromboses in acute coronary syndrome.	Dyspnea, headache. Contraindicated in patients with history of brain hemorrhage.
Antiplatelet agents			
Aspirin Ibuprofen	Inhibits cyclooxygenase. Thus prevents formation of thromboxane A_2 and prostaglandins (which induce platelet aggregation).	Aspirin reduces risk of recurrent transient ischemic attacks or stroke. Reduces risk of myocardial infarction in patients with unstable angina or prior infarction. Both used for antiinflammatory and analgesic purposes.	GI ulceration, bleeding, hemorrhage.
Clopidogrel (Plavix) **Ticlopidine** (Ticlid)	Blocks platelet aggregation by inhibiting ADP receptor	Reduction of atherosclerotic events.	Similar to aspirin, Neutropenia and rare thrombotic thrombocytopenic purpura with ticlopidine.
Cilostazol (Pletal)	Inhibits phosphodiesterase III. Dilates lower extremity blood vessols.	Intermittent claudication.	Headache, heart palpitations.
Dipyridamole (Persantine)	Inhibits phosphodiesterase, increasing cAMP levels to potentiate PGI_2 (platelet aggregation inhibitor). ↑ levels of adenosine (a coronary artery vasodilator) Has few clinical effects alone.	With warfarin, prevents emboli from artificial valves. With aspirin, enhances lifespan of platelets in patients with thrombotic disease.	May worsen angina. Dizziness, headache, syncope, GI disturbances, rash.
Abciximab (ReoPro) **Eptifibatide** (Integrilin) **Tirofiban** (Aggrastat)	Inhibit glycoprotein IIb/IIIa, necessary molecule for platelet aggregation.	Acute coronary syndrome.	Bleeding.
Vorapaxar (Zontivity)	Protease-activated receptor-1 (PAR-1) antagonist	Reduce thrombotic cardiovascular events.	Severe bleeding, potentially life-threatening. Depression.
Thrombolytic agents:			
Streptokinase	Activates plasminogen to plasmin. Plasmin digests fibrin and fibrinogen forming degradation products. These products also act as anticoagulants by inhibiting the formation of fibrin.	To lyse thrombi in ischemic, but not necrotic, coronary arteries after infarction. Pulmonary embolism, deep venous thrombosis, occluded A-V cannula in dialysis patients, and peripheral artery thrombosis.	Bleeding, bruising. Rarely immune oranaphylactic responses even through it is a foreign protein.
Urokinase	" "	" "	" "
Tissue plasminogen activator (TPA)	Binds to fibrin, then activates fibrin-bound plasminogen to plasmin.	To reperfuse coronary arteries that are occluded.	Hematoma at catheterization site.
Alteplase (Activase) **Reteplase** (Retavase) **Tenecteplase** (TNKase)	Recombinant forms of tissue plasminogen activator.	Acute myocardial infarction (both). Ischemic stroke, pulmonary embolism (Alteplase).	Bleeding.
Direct Thrombin Inhibitors			
Argatraban	Blocks circulating and clot-bound thrombin	Alternative to heparin in heparin-induced thrombocytopenia	Bleeding
Bivalirudin (Angiomax)	" "	Alternative to heparin in patients undergoing coronary angioplasty.	" "
Dabigatrin (Pradaxa)	" "	Prevent clots in patients with atrial fibrillation.	" "

PHARMACOKINETICS	DRUG INTERACTIONS	NOTES
PO.	Aspirin reduces efficacy. Increased cardiac toxicity with digoxin.	Ticagrelor binds ADP receptors reversibly. Prasugrel is irreversible.
Well absorbed primarily in upper small intestine. Distributes to CNS. Metabolized in liver, half-life = 15 min.	Increased risk of bleeding with anticoagulants. Increased risk of GI ulceration with alcohol, corticosteroids, phenylbutazone, oxyphenbutazone. Decreases uricosurea effects of probenecid and sulfinpyrazone and diuretic effects of spironolactone. Decreases absorption of tetracycline. Increases plasma levels of methotrexate.	
PO. Metabolized to active drug.	Increased bleeding risk with other antithrombotic agents.	Consider stopping prior to surgical or dental procedures.
PO. Absorption increased by fatty meals.	Levels increased by omeprazole, macrolides diltiazem.	Contraindicated in patients with congestive heart failure.
Pharmacokinetics are not well established.		
IV	Contraindicated in cases of recent bleeding.	Increased bleeding risk with anti-coagulants.
PO. Once daily. Long half-life.	History of stroke, intracranial hemorrhage, bleeding ulcer	Many – see package insert.
In patients with antibodies against streptokinase (resulting from streptococcal infections), half-life is 12 min. In others, half-life = 83 min.	Enhances risk of bleeding caused by aspirin, heparin, or other anticoagulants.	Isolated from Group C beta-hemolytic streptococci
IV. Administered as infusion over many hours.	" "	Currently isolated from cultured human renal cells. Very expensive.
IV infusion. Half-life = 8 min. Metabolized by liver.		
IV		Contraindicated in cases of recent bleeding.
IV	Enhanced risk of bleeding with other antithrombotics	Derivative of the saliva of the medicinal leech *Hirudo medicinalis*
" "	" "	" "
PO.	" "	

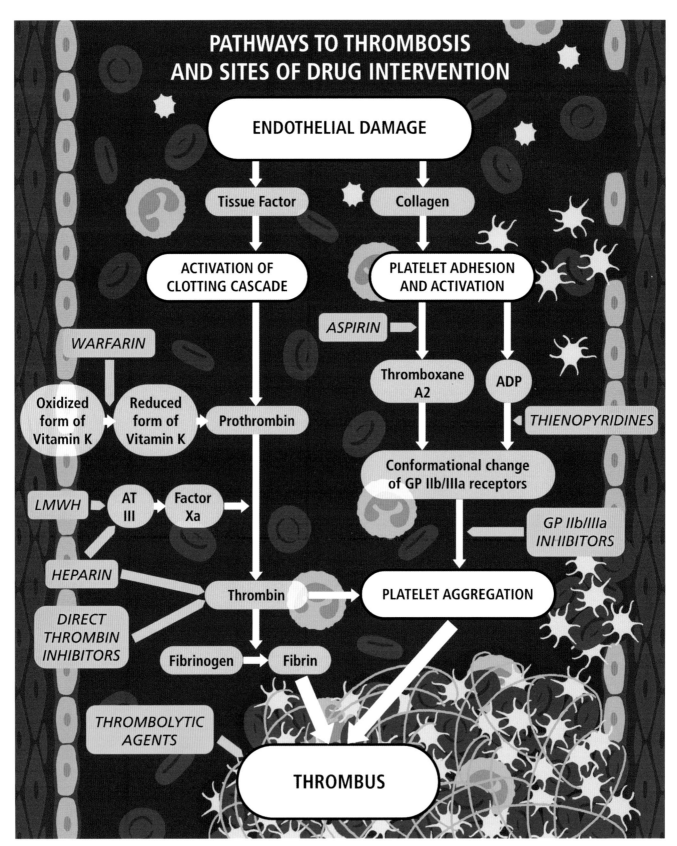

PATHWAYS TO THROMBOSIS AND SITES OF DRUG INTERVENTION

Note: Thienopyridines: clopidogrel, ticlopidine; Glycoprotein (GP) IIb/IIIa inhibitors: abciximab, eptifibatide, tirofiban; Low molecular weight heparin (LMWH): enoxaparin, fragmin; Direct thrombin inhibitors: bivalirudin, lepirudin, argatroban; Thrombolytic agents: tPA, rPA, TNK-tPA; AT III = Antithrombin III; Factor Xa = Activated Factor X; ADP = Adenosine Diphosphate.

Chapter 5 **Respiratory Drugs**

Obstructive Lung Disease

Bronchoconstriction, inflammation and loss of lung elasticity are the three most common processes that result in bronchial obstruction. Therapy for obstructive lung disease is aimed at preventing or reversing these processes.

Bronchoconstriction results from the effects of acetylcholine, histamine, and inflammatory mediators released within the bronchial walls. The vagus nerve releases acetylcholine in response to stimulation of upper airway mucosa by irritants. Acetylcholine also triggers release of pulmonary secretions which further reduce air flow by plugging airways. Sympathomimetics (adrenergic agonists, cholinergic antagonists), methylated xanthines and corticosteroids reverse or reduce bronchoconstriction (Tables 5.1A and 5.1B).

Chronic Inflammation is caused by prolonged exposure to airway irritants such as pollution and cigarette smoke. Bronchiolar inflammation results in narrowed airways, increased secretions, epithelial proliferation, loss of ciliated epithelium and fibrosis. Corticosteroids inhibit the inflammatory response, but their use is at the expense of systemic side effects (Table 5.1B).

Loss of lung elasticity results in terminal bronchiole enlargement, changes in lung compliance and the collapse of airways which are normally tethered open by surrounding lung tissue. It has been suggested that cigarette smoke stimulates proteases and inhibits antiproteases. The relative abundance of proteases degrade normal lung tissue leading to a loss of supportive lung tissue. Specific therapy to reverse or prevent proteolytic destruction of lungs is not readily available.

For diagnostic and treatment purposes, obstructive lung disease is subclassified as either **reactive** airway disease or **chronic** obstructive lung disease (COPD).

Reactive Airway Disease (RAD, asthma): The trachea and bronchi of patients with reactive airway disease are particularly sensitive to stimulants such as cigarette smoke, dust, cold air and allergens. Patients present with wheezing, coughing and chest tightness. Decreased oxygenation of the lungs secondary to tracheobronchial constriction, mucus production, inflammation and edema cause these symptoms.

Therapeutic strategies are discussed below. Hospitalization, oxygen supplementation, nebulized bronchodilator therapy, corticosteroid therapy and occasionally intubation are required for severe episodes.

Chronic Obstructive Pulmonary Disease (COPD): Patients with chronic bronchitis and/or emphysema experience chronic dyspnea as a result of airway obstruction and inflammation. COPD patients complain of persistent cough and dyspnea on exertion. On physical examination, use of accessory respiratory muscles and expiratory wheezing are commonly noted. Expiratory wheezing is due in part to bronchiolar collapse which traps air distal to the constricted site.

Treatment Options

The method of treatment depends on the severity of the episode and the patient's response to previous therapy. Therapeutic options include:

• **Beta-adrenergic agonists** bind to β_2 receptors on bronchial smooth muscle, causing an increase in the biochemical messenger, cyclic AMP (cAMP). Increased levels of cAMP cause relaxation of bronchial muscle cells, resulting in bronchodilation.

β_2-selective agents are preferred to nonselective β-blockers because they are less likely to cause tachycardia (mediated by β_1 receptors). These agents are first line for prophylaxis and treatment of asthma.

• **Corticosteroids** decrease peribronchial inflammation. Inhaled steroids are recommended in conjunction with beta agonists and cromolyn for asthma prophylaxis. Corticosteroid "bursts" (high doses for a few days) are sometimes used when maintenance therapy fails to control asthma.

Table 5.1A Drugs Used in Bronchial Disorders

DRUG	MECHANISM/ACTIONS	INDICATIONS	UNDESIRABLE EFFECTS
Adrenergic Bronchodilators			
Albuterol (e.g., Ventolin, Proventil)	β_2 adrenergic receptor agonist-causes bronchodilation.	Drug of choice for treatment of acute asthma symptoms and to prevent exertion-induced asthma.	Though promoted as a β_2-"selective" agonists, side effects parallel "nonspecific" agonists (vasodilation, tachycardia, CNS stimulation (Table 2.1). Inhalation preparations have fewer side effects.
Metaproterenol (e.g., Alupent)	" "	" "	" "
Terbutaline (e.g., Brethaire)	" "	" "	" "
Formoterol (e.g., Perforomist)	" "	" "	" "
Pirbuterol (Maxair)	" "	" "	" "
Levalbuterol (Xopenex)	" "	" "	" "
Arformoterol (Brovana)	" "	" "	" "
Salmeterol (Serevent)	Long acting $\beta_2 > \beta_1$ agonist.	Chronic treatment of asthma or bronchospasm in adults. Not for acute exacerbations.	Nasopharyngitis, headache, cough.
Epinephrine (e.g., Primatene Mist)	Adrenergic agonist causes bronchodilation (β_2 receptors,) vasoconstriction (α1) and ↓ secretions (α1). More detail in Table 2.1.	Used emergently for severe bronchoconstriction/ vasodilation (anaphylaxis).	Tachycardia, metabolic and GI abnormalities, CNS stimulation (See Table 2.1).
Ephedrine	α β_1 β_2	" "	" "
Isoproterenol (e.g., Isuprel)	β_1 and β_2 agonist. See Table 2.1.	Like epinephrine, but requires prescription.	" "
Indacaterol (Arcapta) **Olodaterol** (Striverdi)	Long-acting adrenergic agonist bronchodilator	Chronic obstructive pulmonary disease (COPD).	Chest pain, cough, troubled breathing.
Anticholinergics			
Ipratropium (Atrovent) **Aclidinium** (Tudorza) **Umeclidinium** (Incruse) **Tiotropium** (Spiriva) **Revefenacin** (Yupelri)	Muscarinic antagonist. Reverses acetylcholine-induced bronchoconstriction.	Bronchospasm associated with COPD in adults.	Few systemic anticholinergic side Effects because these compounds cross into systemic circulation poorly.

- **Cromolyn** is a prophylactic agent. It inhibits the release of mediators from inflammatory cells, such as mast cells. It is used exclusively in asthma.

- **Methylxanthines** increase cAMP and inhibit adenosine-induced bronchoconstriction. Oral theophylline is used for outpatient management of asthma less frequently than in the past. An intravenous bolus of aminophylline, the water-soluble salt of theophylline, produces therapeutic serum levels faster than oral theophylline. Aminophyline is therefore used in acute management.

- **Cholinergic Antagonists** reduce bronchoconstriction and secretions caused by parasympathetic transmission. Ipratroprium bromide is preferred for the treatment of non-asthmatic COPD in adults and is a secondary drug in the treatment of asthma.

Most of these agents are administered by inhalation. Consider improper administration of bronchodilators as an explanation for therapeutic failure.

PHARMACOKINETICS	CONTRAINDICATIONS	DRUG INTERACTIONS	NOTES
[a]Inh: Ons < 15 m, Dur 3–4 h PO: Ons < 30 m, Dur 4–8 h. *Time of onset and duration are most important points of distinction between these drugs.*		MAO inhibitors, tricyclic antidepressants and other sympathomimetics enhance sympathomimetic effects, may induce toxicity. β-blockers inhibit activity.	Bronchodilation severely reduced in hypoxic and acidotic patients. Physician should be consulted if increased frequency required for symptomatic relief.
Inh: Ons < 5 m, Dur 3–4 h PO: Ons 15–30 m, Dur 4 h		" "	" "
SC: Ons 5–15 m, Dur 2–4 h PO and Inh like albuterol.		" "	High first pass metabolism.
Inh: Ons < 5 m, Dur > 4h.		" "	" "
" "		" "	" "
" "		" "	" "
" "		" "	" "
Inh: Ons 20 m, Dur 12 h. Twice a day dosing.		" "	
SC/Inhalation. SC works immediately. Short acting regardless of route of administration.	Hypertension, hyperthyroidism, cerebrovascular insufficiency, glaucoma.	" "	" "
PO: Ons < 10 m, Dur 3–5 h SC: Ons > 30 m, Dur < 1 h IM: Ons 10–20 m, Dur < 1 h IV: immediate, short-acting	" "	" "	
Inhalation/IV/sublingual.	Tachycardia.	" "	Withdrawal may induce reflex bronchoconstriction.
Long acting	Not for acute COPD attack or asthma.	" "	Take daily at same time each day.
Inhalation.	Narrow angle glaucoma, prostatic hypertrophy.	Additive effect with adrenergic agonists.	Also marketed in combination with albuterol.

[a] Abbreviations: Inh = Inhalation, SC = subcutaneous, Ons = onset, Dur = duration, m = minutes, h = hours.

Table 5.1B Drugs Used in Bronchial Disorders (cont.)

DRUG	MECHANISM/ACTION	INDICATIONS	UNDESIRABLE EFFECTS
Bronchodilators – Methylxanthines			
Theophylline (e.g., Theo-Dur)	The mechanism by which methylxanthines dilate bronchioles is unknown. At toxic doses, these agents inhibit phospho-diesterase, the enzyme which breaks down cAMP (the second messenger that mediates adrenergic- induced bronchodilation). Methylxanthines block adenosine receptors which may account for CNS and cardiac stimulation. Methylxanthines also induce diuresis by an unknown mechanism.	Used for maintenance therapy in moderate to severe asthma. Slow onset limits effectiveness in acute situations. Theophylline is being replaced by ipratroprium bromide and/or sympathomimetic agents for non-asthmatic COPD.	Nausea, vomiting, headache, insomnia, tachycardia, dizziness, neuromuscular irritability, seizures. Side effects are dose related ($\uparrow\uparrow$ risk when serum concentration $>$20 µg/ml). Serum levels can be easily monitored.
Aminophylline	" "	IV loading dose for severe, acute bronchoconstriction. (Theophylline cannot be administered IV.)	" "
Corticosteroids			
Systemic (Listed in Table 10.2)	Decrease inflammation and edema in respiratory tract. Enhance activity of sympathomimetics in hypoxic and acidotic states.	Asthma which can not be controlled by sympathomimetics (bronchodilators) alone.	Sodium/water retention and subsequent cardiovascular problems, weakness, osteoporosis, peptic ulcers.
Beclomethasone (e.g., Beclovent) **Budesonide** (Pulmicort) **Fluticasone** (Flovent)	" "	Control the symptoms of asthma	Usually do not induce systemic toxicity. Actions primarily in lungs. Increases risk of oral *Candida albicans* infection (thrush).
Flunisolide (Aerobid) **Mometasone** (Twisthaler) **Ciclesonide** (Zetonna)	" "	" "	" "
Triamcinolone (Azmacort)	" "	Prevent and treat allergy symptoms	" "
Inflammatory Cell Stabilizers			
Cromolyn (Intal) **Nedocromil** (Tilade)	Prevents the release of inflammatory mediators (e.g., histamine) from mast cells, macrophages, neutrophils and eosinophils.	*Prophylaxis* of asthma attacks. Not useful against an ongoing attack.	Minimal side effects such as throat irritation.
Leukotriene Receptor Antagonists			
Zafirlukast (Accolate) **Montelukast** (Singulair)	Competitive antagonist of leukotriene D4 and E4 receptors. Inhibits bronchoconstriction and inflammation.	Prophylaxis and chronic asthma treatment.	Headache, GI distress. Increased respiratory infection in older patients.
Zileuton (Zyflo)	Inhibits 5-lipoxygenase, an enzyme required for leukotriene synthesis.	" "	Headache, GI symptoms. Liver enzyme elevation.
Benralizumab (Fasenra) **Mepolizumab** (Nucala)	Monoclonal antibody that binds interleukin-5 receptor on eosinophils and basophils (which contribute to asthma), leading to natural killer cell-mediated death.	Maintenance asthma therapy. Not for acute asthma exacerbations.	Hypersensitivity (allergic) reaction to drug.
Reslizumab (Cinqair)	" "	" "	" "

PHARMACOKINETICS	CONTRAINDICATIONS	DRUG INTERACTIONS	NOTES
PO/PR. Well absorbed, liver metabolism, kidney excretion. Dozens of standard and long-acting preparations available.	Patients with seizure disorder, cardiovascular disorder or peptic ulcer disease.	Sympathomimetics ↑ risk of heart and CNS toxicity. Cimetidine, oral contraceptives and several antibiotics ↑ half-life of theophylline – thus ↑ toxicity. Phenobarbital and phenytoin induce metabolism of theophylline, thus ↓ half-life. Dehydration results from ↑ diuresis with concurrent use of furosemide.	Warn patients: doubling a dose, even if one is missed, is very dangerous. Intoxication may cause seizures. Treat overdose with ipecac, activated charcoal, and a cathartic.
IV/PO/PR. Increased solubility allows IV administration.	" "	" "	Aminophylline is the water soluble salt of theophylline. It is 79% theophylline.
PO/IV/IM.			Steroids are adjunct agents and should be discontinued as soon as possible.
Inhalation. Rapid inactivation in lungs.	Treatment of status asthmaticus (drug does not adequately relieve symptoms), patients w/systemic fungal infections.		Inhalation agents must not be substituted for systemic steroids without first tapering systemic steroids.
" "	" "		" "
" "	" "		" "
Inhalation. Slow onset of action. Effective prophylaxis may require several weeks of therapy.			May allow patient to reduce maintenance dose of bronchodilators or corticosteroids.
PO. Well absorbed. Peak levels in 3 hours. Inhibits P450.	Not indicated for reversal of bronchospasm in acute asthma attacks.	Theophylline, erythromycin reduce Zafirlukast levels. Phenobarbitol decreases Montelukast.	Efficacy similar to cromolyn.
" "	" "	Increases serum theophylline level	" "
Subcutaneous administration. Very long serum half-life.	Patients with helminthic infection (eosinophils clear helminths).		Do not wean steroids too rapidly after starting this drug.
Intravenous administration			

Table 5.2 Monoclonal Antibodies for Severe Asthma

DRUG	TARGET	DESCRIPTION
Omalizumab	IgE	Monoclonal antibodies are used for severe asthma driven by Type-2 inflammation involving eosinophils or mast cells triggered by TSLP, IL-25, IL-33, IL-4, IL-5 and IL-13. It is important to phenotype the patient to match the drug with the disease driver.
Mepolizumab Reslizumab Benralizumab	IL-5 pathway	" "
Tralokinumab	IL-13	" "
Dupliumab	IL-4Rα	" "
Tezepelumab	TSLP	" "

Table 5.3 Miscellaneous Respiratory Drugs

DRUG	DESCRIPTION
Surfactant Beractant Luciactant Calfactant Paractant	Infant respiratory distress syndrome (IRDS) is caused, in part, by surfactant deficiency. Surfactant decreases surface tension in the lungs, permitting alveoli to open more readily. Exosurf and Survanta are surfactant replacement products administered endotracheally to reduce the incidence and severity of IRDS. Survanta is isolated from bovine lung and supplemented to resemble natural surfactant. Exosurf is a synthetic surfactant analog. Toxicity includes desaturation and bradycardia during administration and risk of pulmonary hemorrhage.
N-Acetylcysteine (e.g., Mucomyst)	Mucolytic agent reduces viscosity of mucous by cleaving protein complexes. Used in patients with chronic bronchopulmonary disease.
Alpha$_1$-Proteinase Inhibitor Roflumilast (Zoryve)	Patients with alpha1 antitrypsin deficiency develop pan acinar emphysema due to degradation of elastin by neutrophil-produced elastase. Alpha$_1$-Proteinase Inhibitor is purified from pooled human plasma and is administered intravenously each week. The primary toxicity is fever.
Palivizumab (Synagis)	A humanized monoclonal antibody targeted against respiratory syncytial virus (RSV). It provides passive immunity for high risk infants (prematurity, bronchopulmonary dysplasia) when given as monthly IM injections during winter and early spring months when RSV infections are prevalent in the community.
Intranasal Steroids **Beclomethasone** (e.g., Becanase) **Budesonide** (Rhinocort) **Ciclesonide** (Omnaris) **Flunisolide** (Nasalide) **Triamcinolone** (Nasacort) **Fluticasone** (Flonase) **Mometasone** (Nasonex)	Inhibit inflammatory cells in nasal mucosa. Reduce symptoms of rhinitis. May increase risk of thrush (oropharyngeal candida) and prevent healing of damaged nasal mucosa.
Antihistamines	Presented in Table 9.7.

Chapter 6 **Gastrointestinal Agents**

Drugs for Stomach Disorders

Helicobacter pylori is a bacterium that causes most cases of gastritis and duodenal ulcer disease. *H. pylori* ulcers are in some cases precancerous. Prior to the identification of *H. pylori* as a causitive agent, peptic ulcers were treated with agents that reduced or neutralized gastric acid.

Current practice utilizes at least two antibiotics with an antisecretory agent and/or bismuth. Although *H. pylori* is readily suppressed by a single antibiotic, monotherapy is suboptimal because it fails to eradicate the organism and leads to selection of resistant organisms. Antibiotics typically used for *H. pylori* disease include **amoxicillin, clarithromycin, metronidazole or tetracycline**. These are reviewed in Chapter 7.

Antisecretory agents include proton pump inhibitors (e.g., omiprazole) and H2 histamine receptor antagonists (e.g., ranitidine) which are described in Table 6.1. These agents reduce gastric acid production and promote mucosal healing. **Bismuth** reduces bacterial adherence to mucosal cells and damages bacterial cell walls. It is also the active ingredient in Pepto-Bismol, an anti-diarrheal agent.

Gastroesophageal Reflux Disease (GERD) and Dysmotility Reflux esophagitis is an inflammation of esophageal mucosa caused by reflux of acidic stomach contents into the esophagus. The underlying defect is usually an incompetent lower esophageal sphincter. The disease is exacerbated by obesity and smoking (nicotine relaxes the lower esophageal sphincter). Nonmedical treatment includes elevation of the head of the bed, avoidance of eating before sleep, loose fitting clothing and surgical procedures that restore the competency of the lower esophageal sphincter.

H_2 histamine-receptor antagonists are effective for short-term treatment of GERD (Table 6.1). Similarly, agents that increase the rate of gastric emptying, inhibit the proton pump of gastric parietal cells, form a protective coat in the stomach or augment endogenous prostaglandins to promote bicarbonate and mucin release are used for GERD, dysmotility, or stomach mucosa protection (Table 6.1).

Antacid salts, available over the counter (e.g., TUMS), provide transient symptomatic relief of gastric acid irritation. Drugs which alter stomach or duodenal pH frequently alter absorption of other oral drugs. Review potential drug interactions before prescribing.

Antidiarrheals

Diarrhea is usually caused by infection, toxins or drugs. Antidiarrheal agents are described in Table 6.2. Several of these drugs are sold over-the-counter and are used more frequently than medically indicated.

Viral or bacterial-induced diarrhea is usually transient and requires primarily a clear liquid diet and increased fluid intake. Antimicrobial therapy may be indicated by the presence of specific pathogens in the stool or fecal leukocytes. Intravenous fluids may be required if dehydration occurs.

Table 6.1 Acid Reducing Agents and Dysmotility Agents

DRUG	MECHANISM/ACTIONS	INDICATIONS	UNDESIRABLE EFFECTS
Amoxacillin Clarithromycin Metronidazole Tetracycline	See chapter 7	*H. pylori* ulcers	See chapter 7
H₂ Histamine Receptor Antagonists:			
Cimetidine (Tagamet)	H₂ Histamine Receptor Antagonist.	Duodenal/gastric ulcer, hypersecretion of acid, GERD.	Well tolerated. Diarrhea, dizziness, rash, headache, confusion, somnolence, decreased libido, impotence, gynecomastia. Rarely, blood dyscrasias, hepatotoxicity and renal toxicity.
Ranitidine (Zantac)	" "	" "	Similar to cimetidine. Possibly less CNS and sexual disturbance than cimetidine.
Famotidine (Pepcid)	" "	" "	" "
Nizatidine (Axid)	" "	Duodenal ulcers, benign gastric ulcers.	" "
Antacids			
Calcium Carbonate	" "	" "	Constipation, hypercalcemia, metabolic alkalosis, hemorrhoids, bleeding anal fissures. Rarely, milk-alkali syndrome (if taken chronically with milk or bicarbonate).
Magnesium Salts	" "	" "	Diarrhea, hypermagnesemia (nausea, vomiting, hyporeflexia, decreased muscle tone).
Na⁺ Citrate	" "	Preferred pre-op antacid.	Horrible taste. Less likely than others to cause aspiration pneumonitis in sedated patients because it is nonparticulate.
Miscellaneous:			
Sucralfate (Carafate)	Sucrose and polyaluminum hydroxide polymerize at low pH to form protective coating.	Prophylaxis and treatment of duodenal ulcers.	Constipation.
Metoclopramide (Reglan)	Increases rate of gastric emptying by unknown mechanism.	Reflux esophagitis, gastroparesis, pre-op gastric emptying.	Diarrhea, constipation, drowsiness, depression. Occasionally, extra-pyramidal side effects due to dopamine antagonism.
Omeprazole (Prilosec) Lansoprazole (Prevacid) Dexlansoprazole (Dexilant) Esomeprazole (Nexium) Pantoprazole (Protonix) Rabeprazole (Aciphex)	Inhibits H⁺/K⁺ATPase (proton pump) of parietal cell. Thus, reduces acid secretion.	Reflux esophagitis, duodenal ulcers, hypersecretory states.	Few side effects. Constipation. Causes gastric carcinoid tumors in rats after prolonged use.
Misoprostol (Cytotec)	Increases HCO₃ and mucin release. Reduces acid secretion.	Prevention of ulcers caused by aspirin and other NSAIDS.	Abortion (uterine contraction), diarrhea, abdominal pain, nausea, flatulence.

CONTRAINDICATIONS	PHARMACOKINETICS	DRUG INTERACTIONS	NOTES
See chapter 7	See chapter 7	See chapter 7	Effective therapy requires at least two antibiotics and an antisecretory agent or bismuth.
Use with caution in patients over 50 years old with kidney or liver failure.	PO/IV/IM. Little plasma protein binding, little metabolism.	Increases concentration of anticoagulants, theophylline, lidocaine, phenytoin, benzodiazepines, nifedipine, propranolol, others by inhibiting liver P450 enzymes. Alters serum level of many other drugs. Consult Drug Index.	
	PO/IV. High first pass metabolism, unchanged drug and metabolites excreted in urine.	Less inhibition of P450 metabolizing enzymes than cimetidine.	
	PO.	No P450 inhibition.	
	PO.	" "	
" "	PO.	Decreases absorption of drugs which are preferentially absorbed at low pHs. Increases gastric absorption of drugs normally absorbed in small intestine.	
Diarrhea, ↓ renal function (result: hypermagnesemia) malabsorption syndrome.	PO. Well absorbed, quickly excreted by kidney	" "	Used with aluminum or calcium antacids to prevent constipation.
Congestive heart failure, hypertension.	PO.	" "	
	PO. 3–5% absorbed.	May interfere with absorption of other drugs, especially fluoroquinoline antibiotics.	Use cautiously in dialysis patients. May increase aluminum concentration.
Elderly patients and children are more susceptible to extrapyramidal effects.	PO/IV/IM. Well absorbed, 50% metabolized in liver, excreted in urine.	Sharply increases risk of hypertension with MAO inhibitors. Increases toxicity of antipsychotics. Reduces absorption of many drugs.	
	PO. Acid labile capsule contains enteric-coated granules, short half-life (1–1.5 hr).	Inhibit cytochrome P450. Omeprazole interacts with warfarin, phenytoin and diazepam.	
Pregnancy.	PO. Prodrug is de-esterified to active acid.		Misoprostol is a prostaglandin E analog.

Parasitic infections are treated with agents described in Table 7.10. Antidiarrheal agents that decrease intestinal motility are contraindicated in parasitic infections and some bacterial infections (e.g., shigellosis) because they suppress expulsion of the organisms.

Drug or toxin-induced diarrhea is best treated by discontinuing the causative agent when possible.

Chronic diarrhea may be due to laxative abuse, lactose intolerance, inflammatory bowel disease, malabsorption syndromes, endocrine disorders, irritable bowel syndrome and other disorders. Treatment with nonspecific antidiarrheal agents such as those listed in Table 6.2 may mask an underlying disorder. Treatment of chronic diarrhea should be aimed at correcting the cause of diarrhea in addition to alleviating the symptoms.

Table 6.2 Antidiarrheal and Inflammatory Bowel Syndrome Agents

DRUG	MECHANISM/ACTIONS	INDICATIONS	UNDESIRABLE EFFECTS
Opiates:			
Diphenoxylate and Atropine (Lomotil)	Diphenoxylate is an agonist at opiate receptors in GI tract and atropine blocks muscarinic receptors. Both actions inhibit peristalsis.	Diarrhea	Few, minor side effects include constipation, abdominal and bowel distention, nausea.
Loperamide (Imodium)	" "	" "	" "
Adsorbents:			
Bismuth Subsalicylate (Pepto-Bismol)	Adsorbs toxins produced by bacteria and other GI irritants.	Diarrhea. Prophylaxis for traveler's diarrhea. Large dose requirements limit utility for long trips.	Impaction.
Kaolin/Pectin (Kaopectate)	Adsorbant and protectant of questionable efficacy.	Diarrhea.	May $\uparrow$ K$^+$ loss or interfere with absorption of drugs and nutrients.
Cholestyramine (Questran)	Absorbs bile salts (which cause diarrhea) and *C. difficile* toxin.	Diarrhea caused by *C.difficile* or bile acids.	Constipation.
Others:			
Anticholinergics	Muscarinic agonists. Inhibit GI secretions and peristalsis.	Diarrhea due to peptic ulcer disease or irritable bowel syndrome.	Decrease memory and concentration, dry mouth, urinary retention, tachycardia.
Corticosteroids	Antiinflammatory agent.	Ulcerative colitis, Crohn's disease, other inflammatory bowel diseases.	See Table 10.6.
Antibiotics	See Antibacterial Agents, Chapter 7.		
Inflammatory Bowel Agents:			
Eluxadoline (Viberzi)	mu-opioid agonist	Inflammatory bowel syndrome with diarrhea	Constipation. Uncommon: pancreatitis
Alosetron (Lotrenox)	Selective 5-HT3 (cation channel) receptor antagonist	Irritable bowel syndrome	GI ischemia, constipation
Mesalamine (5-aminosalicylic acid) **Olsalazine** (Dipentum) **Balsalazide** (Colazal) **Sulfasalazine** (Azulfidine)	Anti inflammatory agents	Inflammatory bowel syndrome and/or ulcerative colitis (see drug monographs) and/or Crohn disease	See drug monographs

Drugs Used to Treat Constipation

A variety of factors including low-fiber, diets, drugs (e.g., anticholinergics, antacids or narcotics), prolonged immobilization and abdominal surgery cause constipation.

Constipation in most nonhospitalized patients can be resolved by increasing the fiber content of their diet or by supplementing the diet with bulk-forming agents.

Rectal administration of laxatives is preferred to oral if there is a question of intestinal obstruction. Agents which stimulate peristalsis should be avoided when obstruction is possible.

Laxative abuse is the most common complication of laxative therapy. Chronic use of laxatives may lead to dependence on such agents for normal bowel movements. Senna, in particular, is dangerous when used chronically because it may damage nerves, resulting in intestinal atony.

CONTRAINDICATIONS	PHARMACOKINETICS	DRUG INTERACTIONS	NOTES
Parasitic or bacterial infections accompanied by fever, obstructive jaundice.	PO.	Potentiate CNS depressants. Increases risk of hypertension with MAO inhibitors. Increases risk of paralytic ileus with antimuscarinics.	
Parasitic or bacterial infections w/ fever.	PO.	None identified.	Treat overdose with naloxone.
Aspirin sensitivity.	PO.	Potentiates oral anticoagulants and hypoglycemics, Reduces uricosuric effects of probenecid and sulfinpyrazone.	
Obstructive bowel lesions, children under 3 years old.	PO.	Decreases absorption of many drugs.	
	PO.	Decreases absorption of many drugs.	Used primarily for its lipid lowering effects (Table 4.8).
Closed angle glaucoma, prostatic hypertrophy, heart disease, obstructive bowel disease.	Consult drug digest for specific agents.	Antacids interfere with absorption.	Specific agents discussed in Table 2.7.
See Table 10.6.	PR. Administered as retention enema.		Corticosteroids discussed in Table 10.6.
	PO.	Antihistamines, antidepressants	
See drug monographs	Various	See drug monographs	See Chapter 9 for more details about anti-inflammatory drugs.

Table 6.3 Laxatives and Cathartics

DRUG	MECHANISM/ACTIONS	UNDESIRABLE EFFECTS	PHARMACOKINETICS
Chronic Idiopathic Constipation Drugs			
Plecanatide (Trulance)	Guanylate cyclase C agonist. Induces cGMP-mediated increase in intestinal fluid.	Diarrhea most common. Dehydration in children.	PO
Prucalopride (Motegrity)	Selective serotonin-4 receptor agonist.	Headache, nausea, abdominal pain, diarrhea.	PO
Opioid Induced Constipation Drugs			
Naldemedine (Symproic)	Mu opioid antagonist.		PO
Bulk Forming Agents			
Psyllium (e.g., Metamucil)	Nondigested plant cell wall absorbs water into feces, thus softening the stool.	Well tolerated. Flatulence, impaction (if bolus is obstructed).	PO. Softens feces in 1–3 days.
Stimulant Laxatives and Cathartics			
Bisacodyl (e.g., Dulcolax) **Senna** (Senokot)	Increases water and electrolytes in feces and increases intestinal motility.	Continuous use may cause severe diarrhea.	PO. Softens feces in 6–8 hrs.
Others			
Saline solutions (e.g., Milk of Magnesia)	Mg^{++} or Na^+ salts are poorly absorbed and thus draw water into the lumen.	Precipitation or exacerbation of cardiac, renal, convulsive disorders or hypocalcemia.	PO. Watery excretion of bowel contents in 1–3 hours.
Polyethylene glycol (MiraLax)	Hyperosmolarity draws water into colon.	Cramps nausea bloating.	PO.
Glycerin	Hyperosmolarity draws water into colon.		PR. Evacuates colon within 15 minutes.
Lactulose	" "	Cramps, flatulence, nausea, vomiting.	PO. Metabolized in intestine to lactate which acts as an osmotic laxative
Mineral oil	Lubricates feces and prevents absorption of water from feces.	Anal leakage and irritation, reduces vitamin absorption.	PO/PR.
Docusate (e.g., Colace)	Improves penetration of water and fat into feces.	Diarrhea, abdominal cramps. Increases absorption of mineral oil (do not use with mineral oil).	PO/PR.

Chapter 7 **Anti-Infective Agents**

An ongoing war rages between the medical community and bacteria. Physicians utilize the latest antibacterial weaponry, while bacteria have only personal protective gear and some basic strategies for intercepting weapons. Nevertheless, because of their sheer number, ability to adapt, and unembarassed penchant for reproducing, bacteria often have the upper hand.

Effective antimicrobial therapy exploits the differences between microbial and eukaryotic cells. Organisms that differ significantly from human cells are easier to selectively kill than those which have few unique properties.

When learning the anti-infective agents, it is useful to group antimicrobials based on their mechanism of action and their structure. The mechanism can provide clues regarding a drug's spectrum and potential side effects. For example, gentamicin, an aminoglycoside, gains access to bacteria by an oxygen-dependent pump and then binds to a ribosomal protein unique to bacteria. Based on this one can predict the antibiotic will fail to enter anaerobic bacteria. In addition, one can see that by blocking the energy dependent transport system or changing the ribosomal protein binding site, the bacteria develops resistance to the drug. Finally, when taught that renal tubule cells actively endocytose the drug during excretion, one can predict that gentamicin might be nephrotoxic.

In addition to the mechanism of action, key issues to consider when learning about antibiotics are:

- Chemistry: Subtle differences in chemical structure can alter spectrum of activity, distribution in the body, toxicity and likelihood of resistance.
- Spectrum of activity: It is useful to generalize "Drug A is generally effective against Gram-positives," but important exceptions must also be learned " . . . but it misses *Enterococcus*."
- Mechanisms of microbial resistance to antibiotics and ways to circumvent resistance.
- Toxicity: Learn the most common side effects as well as the uncommon but severe. Uncommon, mild toxicities can be looked up in the future.
- Administration: Oral vs. parenteral, one vs. three doses daily. These parameters affect patient compliance, frequency of hospitalization and cost.
- Distribution: Drugs must reach microbes to be effective. Know which drugs penetrate the blood brain barrier, joint capsules, the eye, and abscess walls. Know which drugs fail to leave the gastrointestinal system and those that concentrate in the urinary tract.

Following an introduction to therapeutic strategies and commonly encountered microbes, this chapter discusses antibacterial, antiviral, antifungal, and antiprotozoal drugs.

Basic Strategies of Antimicrobial Therapy

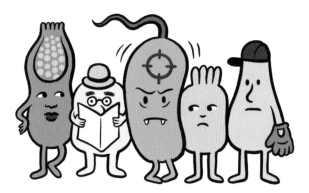

Figure 7.1 Selective toxicity of antibiotics. Bacterial cells differ from normal human cells in that they have cell walls, structurally-different ribosomes, and unique metabolic pathways. Antibiotics are designed to exploit these differences so that bacteria, but not human cells, are damaged.

Don't harm innocent bystanders: The primary goal of antimicrobial therapy is to kill bacteria without harming tissues of the host (Fig. 7.1). Antibiotics exploit the unique features of microbes (cell walls, different ribosomal structures, unique enzymes) absent in eukaryotic cells. Drugs like penicillins have few side effects because they attack bacterial structures that are absent in human cells. These agents have high **selective toxicity** (i.e., good therapeutic index). In contrast, drugs like amphotericin, which attack less unique features in fungi, are toxic to human cells at therapeutic doses (poor selective toxicity).

Follow empiric therapy with focal therapy: The identity and drug-sensitivity of the infecting organism must be determined as rapidly as possible so that rational therapy can be initiated. If the identity of the pathogen is unknown, empiric therapy (best guess) is initiated. The site of infection and Gram stain properties of the organism provide clues to its identity. Rapid identification tests (e.g., latex agglutination) may further confirm the identity. Local susceptibility reports provide information on the susceptibility of pathogens to antibiotics and allow a rational start to antibiotic therapy.

Cultures are the gold standard for identification of microbes. Unfortunately, several days may be required for growth and identification of the organism. **False positive** cultures occur when culture materials become contaminated and when organisms are colonizing (but not infecting) the host. **False negative** cultures occur because of poor sampling technique, prior antibiotic therapy, and inappropriate culture media or techniques.

Empiric therapy should be changed to narrow-spectrum, effective agent(s) when culture and sensitivity results are available.

Sensitivity Determination: The sensitivity of bacteria to various antibiotics is determined by growing cultures in the presence of the antibiotics of interest. The **minimal inhibitory concentration (MIC)** is the concentration of antibiotic which prevents growth of the culture. The **minimal bactericidal concentration (MBC)** is the concentration that kills 99.9% of the inoculum. The **serum bactericidal titer** is the dilution of patient's serum (which contains antibiotic molecules that haven't been distributed to other sites, bound to plasma proteins, metabolized, or excreted) that is capable of killing the pathogen. This provides information on whether the concentration of antibiotics in a given patient is high enough to be effective in body spaces (e.g., joints, meninges) characterized by poor antibiotic permeability.

Keep your empiric therapy arsenal small: Antibiotic therapy often begins before the infectious agent is identified. Each practitioner should thoroughly understand a small number of antibiotics that are frequently used for empiric therapy. The history, infection location and rapid identification tests described above provide clues to the identity of the microbe. The following statements summarize key points about drugs that are frequently used for empiric therapy. If the presumed organisms are:

- **Gram-positives:** Nafcillin (IV) and dicloxacillin (PO) provide excellent coverage of most Gram-positives and are not destroyed by penicillinases. First generation cephalosporins (e.g., cephalexin, cefazolin) are effective against most skin and skin structure infections.

- **Gram-negatives:** Third generation cephalosporins are effective against many Gram-negatives and are not destroyed by cephalosporinases. They penetrate the brain well. Cephalosporins and penicillins may enhance the activity of aminoglycosides against Gram-negatives. The combination of "Amp & Gent" (ampicillin and gentamicin) provides very good coverage of both Gram-positives and Gram-negatives. Trimethoprim-sulfamethoxazole (Bactrim/Septra) is active against most urinary tract infections. Amoxicillin is frequently used for otitis media and other bacterial upper respiratory infections.

- *Pseudomonas:* Ticarcillin or ceftazidime cover most Gram-negatives, including *Pseudomonas*, but fail to treat some Gram-positives. Imipenem and meropenem have good activity against *Pseudomonas*.

- **Anaerobes:** Metronidazole or clindamycin cover most anaerobic bacteria. Mouth anaerobes are adequately covered by penicillin.
- **Mycoplasma:** The macrolides (erythromycin, clarithromycin, azithromycin) treat presumed *Mycoplasma* pneumonia, along with most other organisms that cause community-acquired pneumonia.
- **Systemic fungi:** Amphotericin is the drug of choice for presumed fungemia. Systemic fungal infections occur most frequently in patients that have been on broad spectrum antibiotics that have destroyed their endogenous bacteria, allowing fungal overgrowth.

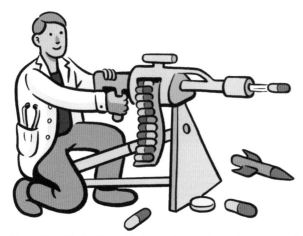

Figure 7.2 *Under the right circumstances, it may be necessary to initiate therapy with several antibiotic agents.*

Sometimes you need more than one antibiotic (Fig. 7.2): Quite often it is advantageous to use multiple drugs to treat an infection. Examples include:

- **Unknown microbe:** If you haven't identified the Gram stain properties of an infectious agent, it is sometimes necessary to treat with antibiotics that cover a broad spectrum of microbes. Often a drug that covers most gram positive organisms and a drug that covers gram negative bacteria are combined. An agent that covers anaerobes or *Pseudomonas* may also be desirable. Single drug therapy can then be instituted when the organism is identified.
- **To prevent resistance:** It is more difficult for bacteria to develop resistance to two drugs with

different mechanisms than to develop resistance to a single agent.
- **To achieve synergy:** The actions of some drugs make other drugs more effective. The classic example is the combination of penicillins or cephalosporins with aminoglycosides. Aminoglycosides work intracellularly, but may have difficulty entering the cell. Penicillins and cephalosporins prevent repair of holes in the bacterial cell wall, making it easier for aminoglycosides to enter.

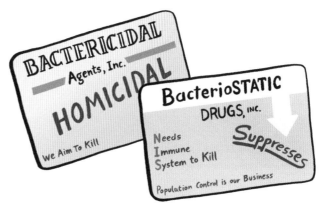

Figure 7.3 *Bacteriostatic drugs require an intact immune system to eradicate an infection.*

Know which drugs kill and which drugs maim (Fig. 7.3): Bactericidal antibiotics kill bacteria (cidal). **Bacteriostatic** agents only inhibit bacterial proliferation while the host's immune system does the killing. Bactericidal agents are necessary for infections in patients with defective immune systems (cancer, AIDS, diabetes) and for overwhelming infections. Patients MUST take their full course of medication. Patient compliance is often poor because it appears that their infection has subsided when in fact it is only suppressed.

Get the drug to the site of infection: The brain, joints, testes, and eye are "protected" sites in the body. Few drugs penetrate the barriers that surround these sites. When treating infections at these sites, one must choose agents that penetrate the barriers and that are active against the infecting organism. Similarly, abscess walls form an effective barrier to antibiotics. Abscesses must be incised and drained.

The Enemies: Gram Positive Cocci

Background: Before the advent of penicillin, Gram-positive cocci were responsible for most known infections. Initially susceptible to basic penicillins, Gram-positive bacteria have developed resistance to basic penicillins and some strains may be resistant to specialized penicillins.

Appearance: Blue & round by microscopy. A peptidoglycan (polypeptide + sugar) cell wall surrounds the bacteria. The impermeability of this wall (compared to Gram-negative bacteria) is responsible for the retention of blue dye during Gram staining. Penicillins, cephalosporins, bacitracin, vancomycin and cycloserine inhibit the synthesis of the peptidoglycan wall.

Common Sites of Invasion: *Staph aureus & Staph epidermidis* inhabit most people's skin and are likely to infect **wounds, surgical sites and indwelling catheters** (may cause infective endocarditis). *Strep pneumoniae* is often the cause of community-acquired **pneumonia** and **adult bacterial meningitis**. "Strep throat" is an infection caused by **Group A beta-hemolytic *Streptococcus***. If untreated, it may elicit an immunologic reaction in the heart, joints and other tissues, known as **rheumatic fever**.

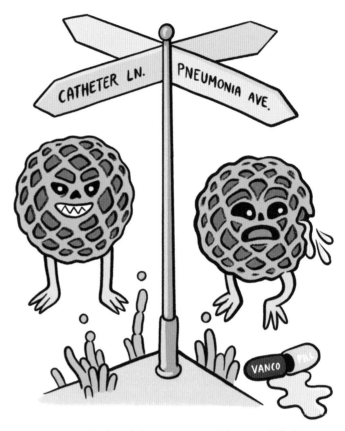

Figure 7.4 Staph. and Strep. are protected by a crosslinked glycoprotein wall. Penicillin, cephalosporins, imipenem, aztreonam and vancomycin prevent construction and repair of the wall.

The Enemies: Anaerobes

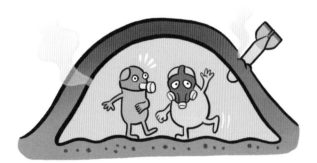

Figure 7.5 Anaerobic bacteria produce foul-smelling infections that are typically encased in an abscess wall. Metronidazole, chloramphenicol and clindamycin are used to treat anaerobic infections, which are typically composed of mixed Gram-positive and Gram-negative organisms.

Background: Common anaerobes include *Bacteroides fragilis, Clostridium difficile* and *Fusobacterium. C. botulinum* and *C. tetani* produce toxins responsible for botulism and tetanus, respectively. Metronidazole, chloramphenicol or clindamycin are effective against anaerobic infections.

Appearance: Mixed Gram-positives and Gram-negatives compose most anaerobic infections. Infections are frequently encased in an abscess wall. Anaerobes produce foul-smelling gas.

Common Sites of Invasion: Anaerobes colonize the mouth, gastrointestinal tract and skin of all persons. Infections develop when anaerobes penetrate poorly oxygenated tissues (e.g., the diabetic foot) or tissues that are normally sterile (e.g., peritoneum). When broad spectrum antibiotics diminish normal bowel flora, *C. difficile* proliferates and releases a toxin that causes pseudomembranous colitis.

The Enemies: Gram-negative Pathogens

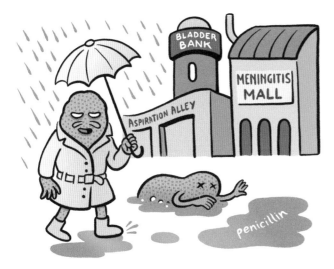

Figure 7.6 Gram negative bacteria. The glycoprotein wall of Gram negatives resembles that of Gram positives. In addition, Gram negatives wear a protective outer coat which is impermeable to penicillin. Ampicillin and amoxicillin however, can penetrate the outer coat and destroy the cell wall. Gram-negatives cause meningitis, pneumonia, bladder infections, otitis media and sinus infections.

Background: Common Gram-negative pathogens can be divided into four groups: 1) Enterics, consisting of those organisms that normally inhabit the GI tract (*Escherichia, Shigella, Salmonella, Klebsiella, Enterobacter, Serratia, Proteus, and others*), 2) *Haemophilus influenzae*, 3) *Neisseria* and 4) *Pseudomonas*. Although rarely a cause of hospital acquired (nosocomial) infections prior to the advent of antibiotics, the enterics are now responsible for most nosocomial infections. Strains resistant to many antibiotics have developed.

Appearance: Enterics and *Haemophilus influenzae* are red and elongated by microscopy (Fig. 7.6). The plasma membrane of Gram-negative bacteria is protected by an adjacent rigid peptidoglycan wall (site of action for penicillins, cephalosporins, etc.) which is encased by an outer membrane. **Penicillins must cross the outer membrane in order to act at the inner cell wall**. The outer membrane is made of lipopolysaccharides interrupted by transmembrane protein pores (which prohibit entry of most penicillins and cephalosporins). **Broad spectrum penicillins and third generation cephalosporins are more hydrophilic** than previous drugs, allowing passage through the selective pores. Even so, some Gram-negative strains are resistant to penicillins because they produce B-lactamases (penicillin-destroying enzymes) that are concentrated in the space between the outer membrane and the cell wall. *Neisseria* are paired red spheres. *Pseudomonas* also has an extracellular polysaccharide slime layer and unipolar flagella.

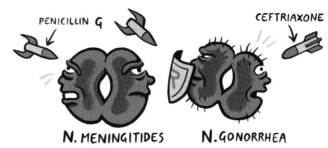

Figure 7.7 *Neisseria meningitides* and *N. gonorrhea* are the only gram negatives that are susceptible to penicillin G and other narrow spectrum penicillins. Ceftriaxone has now replaced penicillin as the drug of choice for *N. gonorrhea* due to the emergence of penicillin-resistant strains.

Common sites of invasion: The **enterics** are responsible for many **urinary tract infections and aspiration pneumonia** due to the proximity of the gastrointestinal tract (their home) to the urethra and the lungs. *Neisseria gonorrhea* is responsible for sexually transmitted **gonorrhea**. *N. meningitidis* and *H. influenzae* both cause **meningitis. H. influenzae** more commonly causes **pneumonia**, particularly in the elderly. *Pseudomonas aeruginosa* is sometimes responsible for **hospital acquired infections**. Pseudomonal infections can occur at any site, particularly in immunocompromised patients. If adequate moisture is available, *Pseudomonas* may colonize any surface in the hospital (including workers) and is resistant to many disinfectants.

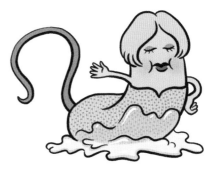

Figure 7.8 *Stella Pseudomonas shows off her slime coat and flagella, which distinguish her from the other gram negatives. She can infect any site in the body and is relatively resistant to most antibacterial agents. Tobramycin or ceftazidime are preferred agents for treating Pseudomonal infections.*

Bactericidal Cell Wall Inhibitors

The agents described in Table 7.1 kill bacteria by preventing synthesis or repair of the cell wall. The cell wall protects bacteria, which are hyperosmolar, and prevents them from absorbing water and exploding.

The mechanism of cell wall synthesis is demonstrated in Figure 7.9. In brief, peptidoglycan chains synthesized in the cytoplasm of bacteria are transferred across the plasma membrane and linked to other peptidoglycan chains. The result is a "chain-link" wall that surrounds the bacteria.

Because human cells lack cell walls, they are generally unaffected by inhibitors of cell wall synthesis. This explains why penicillins and cephalosporins have few side effects.

Bactericidal Cell Wall Inhibitors

• Penicillins (β-lactam drugs)

Penicillin was first isolated from the *Penicillium* mold in 1928. It was effective against a variety of bacteria including most Gram-positive organisms. Excessive use of penicillin led to the development of bacterial resistance (penicillinase production), rendering the drug useless against many strains of bacteria. Nevertheless, it remains an inexpensive and well tolerated drug of choice for several infections.

The pharmacokinetics, spectrum of activity and clinical uses of penicillins are presented in Table 7.2.

Chemistry: Penicillins, cephalosporins, monolactams (aztreonam) and carbapenems (imipenem) all have a beta-lactam ring in the center. Some of these are inactived if the ring is cleaved by β-lactamases (Fig. 7.10, 7.11). Others (e.g., aztreonam, imipenem) are resistant to β-lactamases.

Early penicillin was acid labile and could not be administered orally. It was ineffective against many Gram-negative bacteria and was destroyed by β-lactamases. Each of these limitations has been overcome in newer penicillins due to alterations of the chemical structure or the development of adjunct agents such as probenecid and clavulanic acid. These advances are diagrammed in figures 7.10, 7.11, and 7.12.

Clavulanic acid and probenecid potentiate the actions of penicillins and cephalosporins. Clavulanic acid potentiates penicillins by binding to and inhibiting β-lactamase (Figure 7.11). Augmentin® is the trade name for amoxicillin and clavulanic acid, and Timentin® is the trade name for ticarcillin and clavulanic acid. Pobenecid acts by competing with penicillin for the organic anion transport system, which is the primary route of penicillin excretion (Fig. 7.12). The result is higher serum levels of penicillin.

Table 7.1 Bactericidal Drugs that Work at the Cell Wall

DRUG	MECHANISM	CLINICAL USE	UNDESIRABLE EFFECTS
Penicillins and Cephalosporins	Inhibits crosslinking of cell wall components.	See Table 7.2 and 7.3.	Hypersensitivity. Rare nerve, liver or kidney toxicity.
Vancomycin Dalbavancin Oritavancin Telavancin	Prevents transfer of cell wall precursor from plasma membrane to cell wall.	DOC[1]: Penicillin or methicillin-resistant Staph and Strep infections. Bacteriostatic against Enterococcus. Oral: *C. difficile* colitis	Thrombophlebitis, ototoxicity, nephrotoxicity. "*Red Man Syndrome*" when administered by rapid IV: tachycardia, flushing, parestheslas, hypotension, severe nephrotoxicity.
Bacitracin	Inhibits recycling of the carrier which transports cell wall precursors across the plasma membrane.	Gram-positive organisms infecting skin, eye infections.	Severe nephrotoxicity when administered intramuscularly.
Carbapenem			
Imipenem/ Cilastatin (Primaxin) **Meropenem** (Merrem) **Ertapenem** (Invanz) **Doripenem** (Doribax)	Inhibits crosslinking of cell wall components.	DOC: *Acinetobacter*. Excellent coverage of most Gram-positives and Gram-negatives (including those which produce β-lactamases) and *P. aeruginosa*. May find role in mixed infections.	Similar side effects as penicillins. Despite wide spectrum, imipenem rarely causes sterile bowel. Perhaps due to low concentration of drug in bowel.
Monobactam			
Aztreonam (Azactam)	" "	Excellent coverage of Gram-negatives including *P. aeruginosa*. Not active against Gram-positives.	Similar side effects as penicillins (hypersensitivity, seizures, hepatitis), Injection site pain, GI upset.
Lipopeptides			
Daptomycin	Depolarizes bacterial cell membrane.	Skin infections caused by S. aureus, MRSA, strep spectes, enterococcus (Vanco-sensitive).	Hepatotoxicity, diarrhea, rash.

[1] *Abbreviation: DOC = Drug of Choice*

Allergic Reactions: Penicillin reactions range from skin rashes to anaphylactic shock. The more severe reactions are uncommon, but potentially life-threatening. Some allergic reactions are mediated by IgE antibodies. Alternative antibiotics should be used in patients with a history of reactions even though penicillin allergies are overreported. Skin tests using penicilloylpolylysine and penicillin degradation products provide information about penicillin sensitivity in patients with no history of penicillin use. Virtually all patients who are truly allergic to one form of penicillin will be allergic to other penicillins.

PHARMACOKINETICS

See Tables 7.2 and 7.3 for specifics.

PO/IV. Poor absorption, poor CNS penetration, excreted unchanged by kidney.

Marketed in combination with polymyxin or neomycin as a topical agent.

IM/IV. Imipenem is administered with cilastatin (inactive), which inhibits renal metabolism of imipenem. Renal failure requires dose reduction for both.

IM/IV. Wide distribution including joints, brain, and urine. Decrease dose with renal failure.

IV Excreted by kidney.

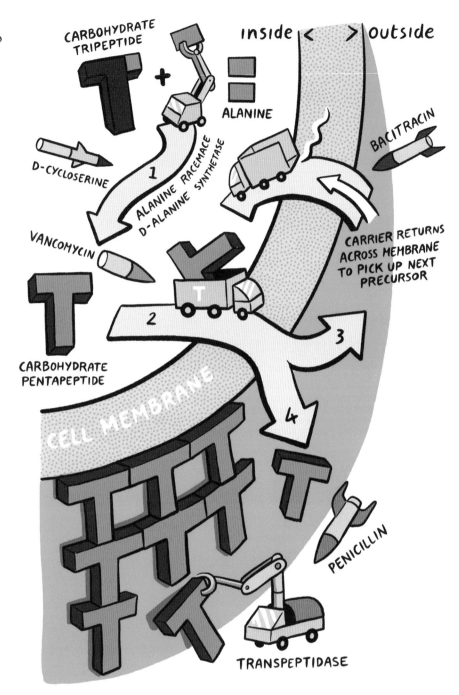

Figure 7.9 Bacterial cell wall synthesis. *1) Alanine molecules are added to a carbohydrate tripeptide to form a "T" shaped cell wall precursor. This reaction is inhibited by D-cycloserine. 2) The precursor is transported across the plasma membrane by a carrier. Vancomycin inhibits the transport process. 3) The transporter is recycled to the inside of the cell to carry other precursors. Bacitracin inhibits this step. 4) The precursor is linked to the existing cell wall structure by transpeptidase. Penicillins, cephalosporins, imipenem and aztreonam inhibit the transpeptidase. Transpeptidase is one of several penicillin binding proteins and is not the only site of penicillin action.*

Figure 7.10 Penicillin Chemistry *Penicillinases inactivate penicillin by cleaving the β-lactam ring. In penicillinase-resistant penicillins, a bulky chemical group prevents entry to the active site of penicillinase, but does not interfere with binding to the bacteria. Narrow spectrum penicillins are unable to pass through the outer membrane of Gram-negative bacteria. Broad spectrum penicillins are more hydrophilic and are thus able to penetrate the aqueous pores of the outer membrane.*

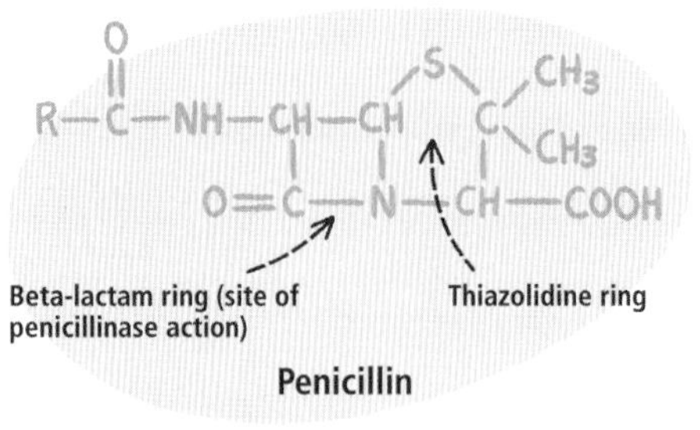

Table 7.2 Penicillins – In Detail

DRUG	MECHANISM	SPECTRUM	DRUG OF CHOICE
Narrow Spectrum, Penicillinase-sensitive			
Penicillin G **Procaine Pen G** **Benzathine Pen G** **Penicillin V**	β-lactam binds penicillin binding proteins (similar structurally to pentapeptide's alanine terminus) and inhibits crosslinking of bacterial cell wall components (Fig. 7.9)	Gram-positive cocci. *Neisseria.* Most mouth anaerobes. **Not effective against** Gram-negative aerobes or β-lactamase producing organisms.	Nonresistant *Staphylococcus* and *Streptococcus, N. meningitidis, B. anthracis, C. tetani, C, perfringens. Listeria. Syphilis.*
Group II Narrow Spectrum, Penicillinase-resistant			
Nafcillin	Bulky side group protects the β-lactam ring from penicillinases. Hydrophobic side group, however, inhibits antibiotic's ability to penetrate gram negative bacteria via hydrophylic porins.	Gram-positive cocci (including β-lactamase producers). Some streptococci. **Not effective against** Gram-negative aerobes.	Penicillinase-producing *Staphylococcus.*
Oxacillin	" "	" "	" "
Dicloxacillin	" "	" "	" "
Group III Broad Spectrum, Aminopenicillins			
Ampicillin	Amino side group makes these agents hydrophilic enough to penetrate the pores in gram negative organisms.	Some Gram-negative and Gram-positive organisms. **Not effective against** β-lactamase-producing organisms.	*Listeria.* *Enterococcus* (if susceptible).
Amoxicillin (Amoxil)	" "	" "	Empiric therapy in otitis media, sinusitis, and pneumonia.
Amoxicillin and Clavulanate (Augmentin)	" " Clavulanate inhibits penicillinases (Fig 7.11).	Gram-negative and Gram-positive and β-lactamase-producing organisms.	*Moraxella (Brahnamella) catarrhalis* and *H. influenza.*
Extended Spectrum, Anti-Pseudomonas Penicillins			
Ticarcillin	Side chain makes it more resistant to β-lactamases from Gram-negative species especially Pseudomonas species.	Gram-negative infections (especially *Pseudomonas*) and aminopenicillin-resistant *Proteus* infections. **Less effective against** Gram-positive penicillinase-producing organisms.	*Pseudomonas*
Piperacillin	" "		Enterobacteria and Gram-positive cocci.
Piperacillin/ Tazobactam	Extended spectrum penicillin combined with beta lactamase inhibitor.	As above plus piperacillin-resistant Gram-negative and Gram-positive penicillinase-producing organisms.	

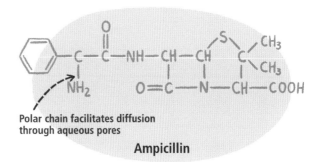

Methicillin

OCH₃ ... OCH₃

Bulky group prevents recognition of methicillin by penicillinases

Ampicillin

Polar chain facilitates diffusion through aqueous pores

PHARMACOKINETICS	SIDE EFFECTS
Pen G IV/IM. Pen V PO (acid stable). Procaine and benzathine prolong half-life. Eliminated by organic acid transfer system in kidney. **Probenecid** competes at this transporter. Can be used to increase penicillin half-life. Distributes to eyes, joints and brain if meninges are inflamed.	Hypersensitivity reactions (anaphalaxis or hemolysis). Rare neurologic toxicity (seizures) due to inhibition of GABA neurotransmission (β-lactam is structurally similar to GABA). Neutropenia. Nephrotoxicity.
IV is preferred route because of low absorption from PO/IM sites. Excreted by liver – high concentration in bile.	" " Severe thrombophlebitis. Liver toxicity with elevated LFTs.
	Like penicillin. Coagulopathy, interstitial nephritis.
PO.	" "
IV/IM/PO.	Diarrhea.
PO.	Diarrhea.
PO.	Diarrhea.
IV.	
PO.	" " Neutropenia and hematologic abnormalities.
IV.	

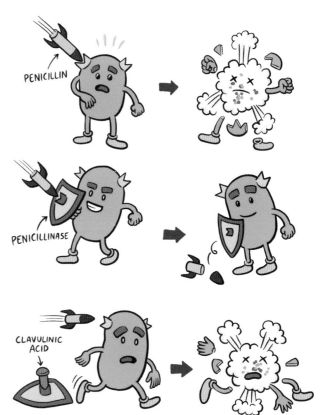

PENICILLIN

PENICILLINASE

CLAVULINIC ACID

Figure 7.11. Penicillinases and penicillinase-resistant penicillins. Top: *Penicillins destroy bacteria after binding to penicillin binding proteins (PBPs).* Middle: *Penicillinases are enzymes produced by bacteria that destroy penicillins by cleaving the beta-lactam ring of the drug. Penicillins are "lured" into the active site because they are chemically similar to penicillin binding proteins.* Bottom: *Clavulanic acid is a "decoy" drug that enhances the activity of penicillins. Clavulanic acid binds to the active sites of penicillinases rendering the enzyme inactive.*

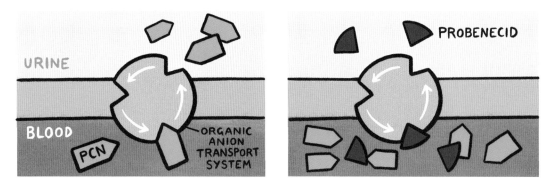

Figure 7.12   Probenecid potentiates the action of penicillins and cephaloporins by competing for excretion at the organic anion transport system (OATS) in the kidney.

Table 7.3 Cephalosporins – In Detail

DRUG	MECHANISM	SPECTRUM	PHARMACOKINETICS
First Generation – Narrow Spectrum, sensitive to Beta Lactamase			
Oral Drugs **Cephalexin** (Keflex) **Cefadroxll** *Parenteral Drugs* **Cefazolin** (Kefzol)	β-lactam binds penicillin binding proteins. Inhibits cell wall synthesis and may in turn activate autolysins. Bacteria develop resistance by reducing drug permeability, mutating penicillin binding proteins and producing β-lactamase and cephalasporinases (clavulanate can circumvent this problem).	Gram-positive cocci except enterococci and Methicillin Resistant *Staph. aureus* (MRSA). Some Gram-negative enterics Not effective against anaerobes Used for surgical prophylaxis and for treating skin or soft tissue infections caused by Staph.or Strep.	Fail to penetrate CSF, Penetrates bone (especially cephazolin). IV drugs achieve adequate tissue and serum levels. Renal excretion of drug and metabolites unless noted. Cephalothin only administered IV because of pain with IM injection.
Second Generation – Broader Gram-negative Activity			
Oral Drugs **Cefaclor** (Ceclor) **Cefprozil** *Oral or Parenteral* **Cefuroxime** (Ceftin) *Parenteral* **Cefoxitin** **Cefotetan**	As above but more resistant to Beta-lactamase activity. Cefoxitin and Cefotetan (cephamycins) are structurally and pharmacologically related to the cephalosporins.	Gram-positive cocci (similar to first generation). Extended Gram-negative activity (*H. flu, Enterobacter, Proteus, Neisseria* species). **None are effective against Pseudomonas.** Used for otitis media, pharyngitis, and sinus, skin, and respiratory infections. Cefuroxime used as single dose therapy for *N. gonorhea.* cefuroxime is more effective than cefazolin in prophylaxis against MRSA wound infections.	Fail to penetrate CSF cefuroxime achieves CSF levels but third generation agents preferred because of greater penetration and more rapid sterilization. Eliminated by kidney.
Later Generation – Broad Spectrum, Resistant to Most Cephalosporinases			
Parenteral **Ceftriaxone** (Rocephin) **Cefotaxime** **Ceftazidime** (Fortaz) **Cefepime** **Ceftaroline** **Cefoperazone** *Oral* **Ceftibuten** **Cefpodoxime** **Cefdinir** **Cefditorin** **Cefixime**	Similar mechanism to first generation cephalosporins; however more resistant to Beta lactamase produced by Gram negative bacteria.	Gram-negative bacilli (resistant to other cephalosporins, penicillins, and aminoglycosides). Variable efficacy against Pseudomonads (ceftazidime, cetipime, and cetoperazone have best coverage). Gram positive cocci (including *Staphylococcus* and nonenteric *Streptococcus*)	Penetrates CSF (except cefoperazone and perhaps cefixime). High levels of ceftriaxone and cefoperazone excreted in bile. Remainder excreted renally. Serum half life – ceftriaxone >> cefoperazone > ceftazidime.

Bactericidal Cell Wall Inhibitors
· Cephalosporins

Cephalosporins share with penicillins a common mechanism, susceptibility to B-lactamases (penicillinases, cephalosporinases) and similar side effects.

Like penicillins, the original "generation" of cephalosporins was most effective against Gram-positive organisms. Chemical modifications increased the effectiveness of subsequent generations against Gram-negatives and reduced their ability to fight Gram-positive infections.

Perhaps the greatest problem with cephalosporins is that their names sound alike. When learning the cephalosporins, concentrate on the commonly used agents first. Each generation has only one preferred oral preparation, usually referred to by the trade names Keflex (cephalexin), Ceclor (cefaclor) and Suprax (cefixime) for 1st, 2nd and 3rd generation, respectively.

Antibiotics that Work Inside the Cell

Up to this point, we have discussed antibiotics that work outside of the bacteria or at its surface. Cell wall inhibitors cannot kill all types of bacteria because some lack cell walls. Other bacteria have unique structures that resist the action or the accumulation of the cell wall inhibitors. Antibiotics that target other vital unique bacterial features are effective in eliminating these infections.

These anti-microbials work within the bacteria and affect the genetic code or protein synthesis. The antibiotics target bacterial structures and enzymes (bacterial ribosomes, bacterial RNA polymerase, DNA gyrase, dyhydrofolate reductase) that although unique to the bacteria, can share homology with host structures. These drugs, therefore, often have poorer selective toxicity than the cell wall inhibitors. The intrabacterial antibiotics have mechanisms of action similar to those used to combat viral, protozoal, and some fungal infections.

The disruption of a microbe's genetic code and the inhibition of DNA replication provide common targets for anti-infectious agents. This can be done by destroying the conformation of the DNA (quinolones/fluoroquinolones), by introducing defective building blocks for DNA synthesis (ddI, ddC, griseofulvin) or by inhibiting enzymes or cofactors necessary for DNA synthesis (sulfonamids, acyclovir, vidarabine). Drugs that target DNA frequently are mutagenic or carcinogenic because they can damage eukaryotic DNA.

The fluoroquinolones are a growing class of antimicrobial agents. The newer quinolones (trovafloxacin, sparfloxacin, and levofloxacin) have improved activity against gram positive organisms. This combined with their excellent gram negative coverage and excellent tissue penetation, has broadened their list of indications to include skin and skin-structure, bone and joint, gastrointestinal, and respiratory infections. Additionally, quinolones can be used for sexually transmitted diseases (gonorrhea and *Chlamydia*).

UNDESIRABLE EFFECTS	NOTES
Hypersensitivity reactions (anaphalaxis, serum sickness). GI disturbances. Rare neurologic toxicity (seizures, confusion) especially with Cefazolin. Hematologic abnormalities; (neutropenia, thrombocytopenia, anemia). Nephrotoxicity and hepatic enzyme abnormalities.	Cross allergenicity between cephalosporin and penicillins occurs in 10% to 15% of patients.
Same as above. Cefaclor associated with high incidence of serum sickness reaction.	Cefotetan (a cephamycin) and Cefpodoxime (an ester prodrug) have improved Gram-negative coverage equivalent to many of the third generation cephalosporins. They are sometimes grouped with the third generation cephalosporins. Cefotetan cefmetazole, and cefoxitin cover *Bacteroides and Clostridium spp.*
Same as first generation cephalosporins. Ceftriaxone associated with acalculous cholestasis and bilirubin displacement from albumin. Use cautiously in neonates and avoid in jaundiced infants.	

Table 7.4 DNA Inhibitors – Fluoroquinolones and Metronidazole

DRUG	ACTIONS-SPECTRUM	UNDESIRABLE EFFECTS	PHARMACOKINETICS
Quinolones			
Nalidixic acid (NegGram)	Blocks a subunit of DNA gyrase. Bactericidal – prevents supercoiling resulting in inhibition of DNA synthesis. Effective against enteric Gram-negative bacteria, but not *Pseudomonas*.	Hypersensitivity reaction, nausea, photosensivity, seizures, headache, dizziness, skin tumors (in mice). Displaces oral anticoagulants from plasma proteins. Causes growth plate arrest in animals – not recommended for children.	PO. This pro-drug is hydroxylated to a bactericidal metabolite which is concentrated in urine. Does not penetrate prostate. >90% plasma protein bound.
Fluoroquinolones			
Norfloxacin (Noroxin)	Disrupts DNA gyrase and DNA topoisomerase activity. Good gram negative coverage.	Drug interactions. Cartilage damage in animal studies. Hence, use in children has been limited.	PO. Reduced bioavailability. Renal elimination. Used primarily for prostatitis or urinary tract infections.
Lomefloxacin (Maxaquin) **Ofloxacin** (Floxin) **Ciprofloxacin** (Cipro)	Disrupts DNA gyrase and DNA topoisomerase activity. Excellent gram negative, some gram positive.	" "	PO. Ciprofloxacin and ofloxacin are also available as IV. Good tissue penetration except CSF. However, ofloxacin has good CSF penetration. Renal elimination.
Moxifloxacin (Avelox)	Does not cover pseudomonas aeruginosa.		PO/IV. Reduce dose with renal impairment.
Gemifloxacin (factive)	Indicated for acute bacterial exacerbation of chronic bronchitis and mild-moderate pneumonia.		PO. Reduce dose with renal impairment.
Delafloxacin	Used to treat skin and skin structure infections		IV/PO
Levofloxacin (Levaquin)	Disrupts DNA gyrase and DNA topoisomerase activity. Excellent gram negative coverage and improved Staph coverage. All treat *Legionella* and *Chlamydia* atypical pneumonia.	" "	PO/IV. Renal elimination. Sparfloxacin is PO only. Good tissue penetration.
Others:			
Metronidazole (Flagyl)	Enters bacteria or protozoan and is activated by reduction of the nitro group. Activated intermediates bind DNA and inhibit its synthesis. Cidal against obligate anaerobes (*Bacteroides, Clostridium, Peptococcus*) and Protozoans (*Entamoeba histolytica, Trichomonas, Giardia*)	Disulfiram-like reaction with alcohol (flushing, vomiting, headache). CNS disturbance (seizures, ataxia, dizziness), nausea, anorexia, bloating, cramping.	PO/IV. Penetrates well into tissues and abcesses, empyemas and CSF. Metabolism is through glucuronidation. Majority of drug is eliminated unmetabolized in the urine.
Nitrofurantoin (Macrodantin)	Mechanism unclear, may damage DNA. Kills many urinary pathogens, but **not** *Pseudomonas, Klebsiella, Proteus, Serratia, Acinetobacter*.	Nausea, vomiting (less so with macrocrystalline formulation), hepatotoxicity, pulmonary fibrosis, neuropathy.	PO. Reduced in liver, excreted by kidney. Reduce dose if renal compromised. Do not administer if creatinine clearance <40 ml/min.
Fidaxomicin (Dificid)	Blocks bacterial RNA polymerase. Indication: *C. difficile* colitis.	Nausea, vomiting, anemia, neutropenia.	PO. Minimally absorbed into bloodstream.

Antimetabolites

The antimetabolites described in Table 7.5 inhibit DNA, RNA and protein production by blocking the folate pathway. Tetrahydrofolate donates single carbon molecules to the synthesis of purines, pyrimidines and some amino acids (methionine, formyl-methionine and serine).

The sulfonamides are structurally similar to para-amino benzoic acid (PABA). Sulfonamides compete with PABA and prevent it from being incorporated into folate (Fig. 7.13). Trimethoprim prevents reduction of dihydrofolate (FAH_2) to tetrahydrofolate (FAH_4) by binding to and inhibiting dihydrofolate reductase (Fig. 7.13). Human cells are spared from this reaction because trimethoprim has very low affinity for human dihydrofolate reductase.

The ability to achieve therapeutic levels of most sulfonamides is limited by precipitation in urine. This problem is circumvented by combining agents. Therapeutic doses of the combination can be achieved with nonprecipitating concentrations of individual drugs.

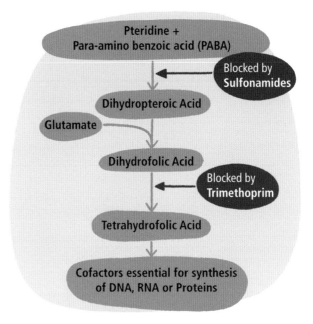

Figure 7.13   *Sites of Antimetabolite Action*

Table 7.5 Sulfonamides and Other Antimetabolites

DRUG	SPECTRUM-USE	UNDESIRABLE EFFECTS	RESISTANCE-KINETICS
Sulfadiazine	Covers both Gram-positives and Gram-negatives. Used for treatment of uncomplicated urinary tract infections, nocardiasis, chancroid, prophylaxis against rheumatic fever. Combined with pyrimethamine for treatment of Toxoplasmosis. Sulfapyridine used for *Dermatitis herpetiformis*.	Bone marrow depression, renal toxicity, photosensitivity, hemolysis, hepatotoxicity, hypersensitivity (fever/rash) Stevens-Johnson Syndrome (serum sickness). Kernicterus – sulfas compete with bilirubin for albumin sites. Resulting elevated free bilirubin is deposited in brain nuclei.	Bacteria which utilize exogenous folic acid are resistant to sulfonamides. PO. Readily penetrates CNS, joints, eye. Precipitates in acidic urine. Encourage fluids to prevent renal stone formation. Major metabolite is acetylated.
Sulfisoxazole (Gantrisin)	" " Prophylaxis of recurrent otitis media and UTI.	" "	" " Higher urine solubility than other sulfonamides.
Trimethoprim/ Sulfamethox-azole (TMP/SMZ, Septra, Bactrim)	Enteric Gram-negatives (*Proteus, E. coli, Klebsiella, Enterobacter*), *H. influenzae, Shigella, Serratia, Salmonella, Pneumocystis carinii*. Inexpensive, effective choice for urinary tract infections, acute otitis media, traveler's diarrhea. Used for *Pneumocysitis carinii* prophylaxis/treatment in immunocompromised hosts.	" "	" " PO/IV. Intermediate urine solubility. High plasma protein binding.

Table 7.6 Inhibitors of Protein Synthesis

DRUG	MECHANISM	RESISTANCE	SPECTRUM OF ACTIVITY
Aminoglycosides (Bactericidal)			
Gentamicin **Tobramycin** **Kanamycin** **Streptomycin** **Plazomicin**	Binds at the 30s/50s subunit interface results in abnormal reading of mRNA and defective bacterial proteins (Fig 7.14). Concentrated in bacterial cytoplasm by energy (oxygen) dependent protein transport.	Mutation of binding sites Inhibition of transport and permeability of drug. * Bacterial enzymatic inactivation of aminoglycoside.	Aerobic and facultative Gram-negative bacilli. Anaerobic bacteria are resistant because transport into bacteria is oxygen dependent.
Amikacin	" "	Has different enzyme resistance profile than gentamicin/tobramycin. * Bacterial impermeability.	" "
Agents that bind to the 50s ribosomal subunit (Bacteristatic)			
Chloramphenicol (e.g., Chloromycetin)	Reversibly binds 50s subunit Preventing aminoacyl end of tRNA from associating with peptidyl transferase (Fig 7.14).	R-tactors code for acetyl transferases which inactivate the drug.	Excellent coverage of most Gram-positives and Gram-negatives, including anaerobes.
Linezolid (Zyvox) **Tedizolid** (Sivextro)	Binds to 50s subunit.		Gram-positive organisms.
Macrolides			
Erythromycin (e.g., E.E.S.)	Prevents translocation of poly-peptide chain by binding to the P site of the ribosomal 50s subunit (Fig. 7.14).	Mutation of binding site by methylation.	Bacteria lacking cell walls (*mycoplasma, legionella, chlamydia*). Most Gram positive aerobes. Gram negative aerobes **except** *Campylobacter, Pasteurella,* some *H. influenza*. Poor anaerobic agent.
Clarithromycin (Biaxin)	" "	" "	As above. Also *Mycobacterium avium intracellulare.* *H. Flu* and some anaerobes.
Azithromycin (Zithromax)	" "	" "	Similar to erythromycin and anaerobic coverage similar to clarithromycin.
Ketolides			
Telithromycin (Ketek)	Binds to 50s subunit		*S. pneumoniae, H. influenza, M. catarrhalis.*
Lincosamides			
Clindamycin (Cleocin) **Lincomycin** (Lincocin)	Binds to 50s ribosomal subunit and prevents chain elongation by blocking transpeptidation (Fig. 7.14).	Alteration of ribosome binding site. Enzymatic inactivation of drug.	Covers Gram-positives and most anaerobes.
Agents that bind to the 30s ribosomal subunit (Bacteristatic)			
Tetracycline **Doxycycline** **Minocycline** **Demeclocycline** **Omadacycline** **Oxytetracycline**	Inhibits protein synthesis. Binds to 30s subunit blocking amino acid-linked tRNA from binding to the 'A' site of the ribosome (Fig. 7.14).	R-factor codes for proteins which transport drug out of cell.	Most *Staphylococcus* and *Strepto-coccus* strains, enterics, mycoplasma, spirochetes, rickettsiae, *Neisseria gonorrhoeae.* Doxycycline approved for malaria prophylaxis.
Tigecycline (Tygacil)	" "		Broad gram-negative and positive activity.

INDICATIONS	UNDESIRABLE EFFECTS	PHARMACOKINETICS	NOTES
DOC: *Enterobacter, E. Coli, K. pneumoniae, Proteus, Serratia, Pseudomonas.*	Nephrotoxicity (assoc. with high troughs). Ototoxicity (assoc. with high peaks).	Slow IV or IM. Not distributed to CNS or eyes. Excreted unchanged in kidney – reduce dose with renal failure.	
Often reserved for Gram-negative infections resistant to other aminoglycosides.	" "	" "	
DOC: *Salmonella typhosa* (typhoid fever), *H. flu* meningitis or epiglottitis. Some physicians/ institutions hesitate to use chloramphenicol due to risk of aplastic anemia.)	Reversible bone marrow supres-sion (binds mitochondrial ribo-somes 50s subunit in bone marrow) or irreversible idiosyncratic aplastic anemia. Gray syndrome (See Notes).	PO/IV Crosses blood brain barrier. Conjugated with glucuronide in liver. Kidney excretion. Decrease dose with liver or kidney disease. Inhibits aminoglycoside transport into bacteria.	*Gray syndrome – toxic levels of drug in newborns unable to conjugate drug. Symptoms: abdominal distention, vomiting, pallid cyanosis, hypothermia, collapse, death (40%).
DOC: Vancomycin resistant gram positive organisms.		Synercid®-IV. Linezoild-IV/PO.	
DOC: *Mycoplasma pneumonia*, neonate with *Chlamydia* pneumonia, Pertussis. **Dirythromycin** used for upper respiratory infections with M catarrhalis, S. pneumoniae.	GI upset. Ilosone prep may cause cholestatic hepatitis. Injections painful due to venodestruction. Increases plasma level of many drugs. Toxicity may result when coadministered w/ theophylline, anticoagulants, carbamazepine.	PO/IV (Erythromycin). Acid labile – take on empty stomach. Concentrated in liver, excreted in bile (active). May pass through inflamed meninges. **Dirythromycin** is a prodrug converted to erythromy-cylamine.	Administer with caution in patients with liver disease or on medication metabolized by P-450 system. Prolonged QT and other arrhythmias possible if patient on terfenidine.
Mycoplasma, Strep throat, upper respiratory infections due to susceptible bacteria, Staph. skiin infections.	Similar to Erythromycin GI upset (less frequently than erythromycin), headache.	PO. Metabolized to active drug by liver.	
Same as clarithromycin plus uncomplicated *Chlamydia* infections.	GI upset (less frequently than erythromycin), abdominal pain.	PO/IV. Take on empty stomach. Long half-life permits once daily dosing. Unmetabolized, excreted in bile.	
Bacterial exacerbation of bronchitis, mild-moderate pneumonia, sinusitis.	Exacerbation of myasthenia gravis. Hepatotoxicity.	PO. Once daily.	
Clindamycin is drug of choice for severe anaerobic GI infections. Also used for *B. fragilis* and *Staph.* infections.	Abdominal cramps, diarrhea, reversible elevation of liver enzymes and GI upset. *Pseudomembranous colitis* seen with any antibiotic but classically associated with clindamycin.	Clindamycin: PO/IV. Hepatic and renal excretion. Reduce dose with impaired liver function. Does not penetrate CSF. Is actively transported into abcesses.	Normal gut bacteria are killed by these drugs. *C. difficile* is resistant and overgrowth/toxin release may follow, causing pseudo-membranous colitis.
Used for acne and chlamydial infections. Also for Borrelia Burgdorferi (Lyme Disease).	GI distress, reversible nephrotoxicity, hepatotoxicity, photosensitivity, dental staining (not used in pre-pubertal children) increased intracranial pressure (rare).	PO. Strong chelator – don't give with milk, antacid, Ca^{++} or Fe^{++}. No CSF penetration. Concentrated by liver, enterohepatic circulation. Excreted in urine and feces.	Combinations with nystatin not effective. Use doxycycline in patients with renal disorders (less nephrotoxic).
Bacteria that are resistant to tetracyclines, methicillin resistant staph, vancomycin resistant enterococci.	Nausea.	IV only.	

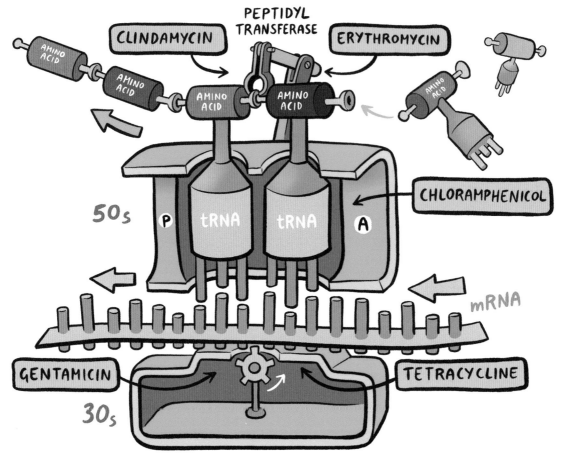

Figure 7.14 Sites of bacterial protein synthesis inhibition. *Bacterial ribosomes exhibit sites that are distinct from human ribosomes. Gentamicin binds at the 30s/50s interface and interfers with mRNA reading. Chloramphenicol, erythromycin and clindamycin bind to the 50s subunit to prevent peptide chain elongation. Tetracycline binds to the 30s subunit which prevents tRNA from binding to the "A" site of the ribosome.*

Protein Synthesis Inhibitors

Bacteria, like eukaryotic cells, must synthesize proteins in order to survive. These proteins provide structural integrity and enable bacterial energy production. Protein synthesis is critical to a micro-organism during replication when new structural proteins and enzymes are essential for progeny. Anti-microbials target several steps in protein synthesis. Some of the drugs can kill but more often they only inhibit reproduction and rely on the immune system to kill the organism. The first step in protein synthesis consists of copying the mRNA code from a DNA blueprint. Rifampin inhibits RNA Polymerase and destroys the code for protein synthesis while the sulfonamides and anti-metabolies block cofactors necessary for RNA and protein synthesis.

After the mRNA code is created it travels to the cytoplasm where ribosomes translate the code into a polypeptide. Other anti-microbials (aminoglycosides, chloramphenicol, erythromycin, tetracycline) target the actual factory (50s subunit of the 70s ribosome) that synthesizes the protein from the mRNA (Fig 7.14). The bacterial ribosomes differ from mammalian ribosomes.

They have different molecular weight (70s vs. 80s), and bind antibiotics preferentially. The mitochondria within the eukaryotic cells contain similar ribosomes to the bacteria.

High exposure to some of these drugs can damaged mammalian tissue by inhibiting this energy producing organelle. Similarly, some of the drugs are less selective for the bacterial ribosomes and can bind to the 80s eukaryotic ribosome and damage host tissue. Rapidly dividing cells, (GI mucosa, skin, bone marrow) and cells in tissues exposed to higher levels of the drug (kidney, liver) manifest the greatest toxicities from these agents.

Mycobacteria

Tuberculosis (TB) and leprosy are the best known mycobacterial diseases. The development of antibiotics changed tuberculosis from a debilitating/fatal illness to one that was readily controlled with oral medications. The prevalence declined until the 1980s, but is now rapidly increasing, particularly among immunodeficient individuals. The organisms are increasingly resistant to multiple antimicrobials.

Mycobacteria are rod-shaped bacilli that stain weakly gram positive. They are called "acid fast" bacilli because they retain dye even when washed with acid alcohol.

Mycobacteria infect mononuclear phagocytes, where they may live for years as intracellular parasites. Fulminant mycobacterial infections develop when the host's immune response is compromised. Thus patients with AIDS and alcohol addiction are particularly susceptible.

Tuberculosis often presents with pulmonary symptoms, but may involve lymph nodes, bones, skin, genitourinary tract and meninges.

Treatment consists of several drugs because resistance develops to single agent therapy. In addition to the emergence of antibiotics resistance, treatment of mycobacteria presents unique problems due to 1) slow growth rate reduces efficacy of antibiotics that prevent rapid synthesis of proteins and DNA, 2) the cell wall is not susceptible to classic cell wall inhibitors, 3) infections may be walled off in tubercles which reduce antibiotic penetration, 4) infections occur frequently in immunocompromised hosts which reduces the utility of bacteriostatic antibiotics (rely on intact host immunity).

Treatment guidelines continue to be revised as multi-drug resistance increases. Prophylactic treatment is recommended for asymptomatic patients that develop skin test positivity and for young (< 4 years) or immunocompromised patients that are exposed to an infectious case of tuberculosis.

Atypical (nontuberculous) mycobacteria: *M. avium-intracellulare* infects patients with chronic pulmonary

Table 7.7 Antituberculosis Drugs

DRUG	MECHANISM	UNDESIRABLE EFFECTS	PHARMACOKINETICS
Isoniazid	Inhibits mycolic acid synthesis in wall of *Mycobacterium tuberculosis*. Bactericidal.	Peripheral neuropathies (can prevent by pretreating with pyridoxine), hepatitis, hepatotoxicity.	PO. Widely distributed. N-acetylated, thus, slow acetylators have greater toxicity. Kidney excretion.
Rifampin Rifapentine	Blocks β unit of bacterial RNA polymerase. Stops bacterial RNA synthesis. Bactericidal.	Secretions (urine, sweat) turn red. Hepatitis (especially in alcoholics), flu symptoms.Induces P450 enzymes, increasing the metabolism of oral contraceptives and other drugs.	PO. Widely distributed – penetrates CNS. Hepatic excretion.
Rifabutin	Synthetic rifamycin with improved activity against rifampin resistant strains of *M. avium.* (in vitro & mouse data).	Similar to Rifampin	PO. Wide distribution. Longer duration of action.
Streptomycin Kanamycin	Inhibits protein synthesis by binding 30s/50s ribosome site. Bactericidal	Vestibular toxicity > nephrotoxicity Rapid resistance by mutation of ribosomal binding site.	IM. Widely distributed – does not penetrate CSF. Poor intracellular penetration. Renally excreted.
Capreomycin	Similar to above. Bactericidal	Ototoxicity and nephrotoxicity.	IM. Excreted renally.
Para-aminosalicylic Acid	Structurally related to sulfonamides – inhibits folate synthesis. Bacteriostatic	Mono-like symptoms, severe GI intolerance and Hypersensitivity lead to poor compliance.	PO. Renal excretion of active metabolites.
Ethambutol	Inhibits mycolic acid synthesis in bacterial cell wall (mechanism not comfirmed) Bacteriostatic	Reversible retrobulbar neuritis. Loss of central vision. Patients must have baseline ophthalmologic exam prior to treatment.	PO. Wide distribution. Reaches 50% concentration in CNS. Concentrated in tubercles.
Cycloserine (Seromycin)	D-alanine analog that inhibits cell wall synthesis. Bacteriostatic.	Allergic dermatitis, CNS toxicity	PO.
Ethionamide (Trecator)	Inhibits peptide synthesis.	Depression, seizures, neuropathy.	PO.
Quinolones	See table 7.4		PO.
Bedaquiline	Blocks mycobacteria proton pump for ATP.	Nausea, vomiting, rash, cardiac/liver/kidney tox.	PO. Avoid administration with rifamycins.

disease and may become fulminant in AIDS patients. Atypical mycobacteria are treated with combination chemotherapy or in some cases, surgery. Because drug resistance is more common in nontuberculous mycobacterial infections than in TB, the susceptibility of the microbe must be determined early.

Antiviral Therapy

Viruses are obligate intracellular parasites composed of either DNA or RNA wrapped in a protein nucleocapsid. Some viruses produce a glycoprotein envelope that surrounds the nucleocapsid. Viruses shed their capsid after invading a host cell. The host cell then synthesizes new viruses using the message encoded by the viral DNA or RNA.

Viral infections are diagnosed by clinical criteria, culture, fluorescent antibody testing, polymerase chain reaction, or serology. Clinically important viral infections include:

- Herpes Family Viruses cause genital and oral herpes, Varicella (chicken pox), and uncommon but severe infections like Herpes encephalitis. Acyclovir is treatment of choice.

- Cytomegalovirus (CMV) is problematic in transplant patients, AIDS patients and other immunosuppressed individuals. Intravenous ganciclovir therapy for CMV infections requires careful monitoring for granulocytopenia and thrombocytopenia.

- Influenza virus infections may be fatal in the elderly or immunocompromised. Amantadine prevents influenza when used prophylactically and reduces the severity of symptoms in infected individuals. Rimantidine is a related drug that has been approved for use in children.

- Respiratory syncytial virus (RSV) causes bronchiolitis in children. RSV usually resolves with supportive treatment. Ribavirin is recommended in children who are at risk for cardiopulmonary complications.

- Human immunodeficiency virus (HIV) is discussed on the next page.

Table 7.8A Antiviral Drugs – DNA and RNA Viruses

DRUG	MECHANISM AND VIRAL SELECTIVITY	CLINICAL USE
Acyclovir (Zovirax) **Valacyclovir** (Valtrex)	Metabolized by thymidine kinase and other enzymes to triphosphate analog which inhibits DNA polymerase and incorporates into viral DNA. Binds to viral thymidine kinase with higher affinity than it binds to mammalian thymidine kinase.	Herpes simplex I and II and *Varicella zoster* virus.
Penciclovir (Denavir)	" "	Topical HSV (coldsores).
Famciclovir (Famvir)	Phosphorylated by viral thymidine kinase to penciclovir triphosphate which inhibits DNA polymerase in HSV.	Shortens duration of herpes zoster and genital herpes.
Ganciclovir (Cytovene) **Valganciclovir** (Valcyte)	Metabolized by thymidine kinase and other enzymes to triphosphate form which inhibits DNA polymerase and incorporates into viral DNA. Preferentially phosphorylated to active drug in CMV-infected mammalian cells.	Cytomegalovirus retinitis and severe systemic CMV infections in immunocompromised hosts.
Foscarnet (Foscavir)	Analog of pyrophosphate. Competes for pyrophosphate site in viral, but not human, DNA polymerase and reverse transcriptase.	Cytomegalovirus retinitis in immunocompromised patients. Acyclovir-resistant HSV infections.
Amantadine (e.g., Symmetrel)	Prevents virus from entering susceptible cells.	Treatment/prophylaxis of influenza A in the elderly and patients with cardiopulmonary dysfunction.
Rimantadine (Flumadine)	Analog of amantadine uncertain mechanism but appears to inhibit viral uncoating.	" " Approved for prophylaxis in children.
Ribavirin (Virazole)	Unknown mechanism.	Hospitalized children with respiratory syncytial virus (RSV) who are at risk for cardiopulmonary complications.
Zanamivir (Relenza)	Inhibits influenza virus neuraminidase.	Treatment of influenza virus infection.
Oseltamivir (Tamiflu)	Analog of adenosine monophosphate	Influenza
Baloxavir (Xofluza)	Inhibits endonuclease activity of the influenza polymerase acipolymerase acidic protein	Influenza

Table 7.8B Antiviral Drugs – Hepatitis

Hepatitis B Agents

Adefovir (Hepsera) **Entecavir** (Baraclude) **Tenofovir** (Viread) **Lamivudine** (Epivir)	Nucleoside analog to control (not cure) chronic hepatitis B. Hepatitis B infection may be exacerbated when drug is discontinued. HIV testing should be offered to all candidates prior to initiating drug to avoid inducing HIV drug resistance in infected patients. Renal dysfunction associated with drug-induced nephrotoxicity. Lactic acidosis and liver damage are potentially severe side effects.
PegInterferon Alfa 2A (Pegasys)	Induces immune activity against hepatitis B.

Chronic Hepatitis C - Agents are used in combination. Please refer to hcvguidelines.org

Sofosbuvir (Sovaldi) **Dasabuvir**	**Nucleotide analog HCV NS5B polymerase inhibitor.**
Paritaprevir Grazoprevir	**HCV NS3/4A protease inhibitors.** Often used in combination products.
Ledipasvir Ombitasvir	**HCV NS5A protease inhibitors.** Ledipasvir, ombitasvir and elbasvir are approved in combination with other hepatitis C drugs and are not approved as single agents.
Combination products	Brand names of current combination therapies include: Harvoni, Viekira Pak, Zepatier, Technivie, Epclusa, Vosevi, Mavyret.

VIRAL RESISTANCE	UNDESIRABLE EFFECTS	PHARMACOKINETICS	NOTES
Resistant strains produce abnormal thymidine kinase or DNA polymerase.	Skin irritation and burning. Crystalline nephropathy if drug is infused rapidly. Nausea, headache.	IV/PO. Administer slowly. CNS level = 50% of serum level. Decrease dose with kidney dysfunction. Poor bioavailability.	Valacyclovir has slightly better oral absorption.
		Topical	
	Minimal toxicity. Headache.	PO. Decrease dose with renal dysfunction.	
Some resistant strains lack thymidine kinase. Cannot activate drug.	Granulocytopenia, anemia, thrombocytopenia. Renal dysfunction.	IV/PO. Excreted unchanged in urine. Decrease dose with renal dysfunction.	Do not coadminister zidovudine (granulocytopenia) or imipenem-cilastatin (seizures).
Because drug does not require phosphorylation, it is active against thymidine kinase-deficient strains.	Renal toxicity (frequent), seizures, hypocalcemia, fever, anemia, diarrhea, nausea, many others.	IV. >80% excreted unchanged in urine. CSF penetration variable. Reduce dose with renal dysfunction.	Deposited in bone and teeth. Hydrate patient during therapy to protect kidneys.
	Depression, CNS toxicity, congestive heart failure, orthostatic hypotension, urinary retention.	PO. Excreted unmetabolized.	
	Fewer CNS side effects, but still risk of seizures.	PO. Prolonged elimination w/renal or hepatic dysfunction.	
	Decreased pulmonary function. Teratogenic in animal studies.	Aerosol administration. Absorbed systemically.	
	Minimal toxicity.	Inhalation.	
		PO	
	Minimal side effects	PO	

Antiretroviral Therapy

The greatest barrier to effective anti-HIV therapy is the emergence of drug resistant strains. Human immunodeficiency virus develops drug resistance by mutating the enzymes that are targeted by antiviral agents. Retroviral reverse transcriptase has low transcription fidelity, so basepair substitutions are common. These mutations translate into amino acid substitutions which, if located in the drug-binding pocket, may reduce the affinity of the enzyme for the drug without diminishing the enzyme activity.

Because of drug resistance, monotherapy is seldom used for treating AIDS patients. More often, when therapy is initiated, multiple agents with different viral targets are used. These multidrug "cocktails" are analogous to combination chemotherapy used for cancer patients.

There are currently three categories of anti-HIV drugs: nucleoside analogs, non-nucleoside reverse transcriptase inhibitors and protease inhibitors (Table 7.8A). By combining medicines from all three mechanistic categories into a single fixed-dose pill that is taken once a day, pharmaceutical companies have made strides toward converting HIV into a chronic illness. This is due to the fact that it is difficult for the HIV virus to simultaneously develop resistance to three or more drugs and because patient compliance in taking medicine is higher for once a day dosing compared to multiple drugs multiple times per day.

Table 7.8C Antiviral Drugs – HIV/Retroviruses

DRUG	MECHANISM AND VIRAL SELECTIVITY	CLINICAL USE
Maraviroc (Selzentry)	**Blocks CCR5 receptors,** blocks CCR5-tropic HIV from entering cells.	CCR5-tropic HIV, as part of combination therapy.
Taltegravir (Isentress) **Dolutegravir** (Tivicay) **Raltegravir** (Isentress) **Cabotegravir** (Apretude)	**Blocks integrase,** the enzyme that integrates viral DNA into the host genome. Integrase is necessary for viral replication.	HIV, as part of combination therapy.
Zidovudine (Retrovir) **Emtricitabine** (Emtriva) **Lamivudine** (Epivir) **Abacavir** (Ziagen) **Tenofovir** (Viread)	**Nucleoside HIV Reverse Transcriptase Inhibitors.**	HIV in combination therapy Zidovudine is used in the prevention of maternal-fetal transmission of HIV.
Doravirine (Pifeltro) **Nevirapine** (Viramune) **Efavirenz** (Sustiva) **Etravirine** (Intelence) **Rilpivirine** (Edurant)	**Non-nucleoside inhibitors of HIV reverse transcriptase.**	HIV. Never as monotherapy due to rapid development of resistance.
Ritonavir (Norvir) **Fosamprenavir** (Lexiva) **Atazanavir** (Reyataz) **Tipranavir** (Aptivus) **Darunavir** (Prezista)	**Protease inhibitor.** Protease is an enzyme necessary for cleaving the gag-pol precurser. Results in immature virus formation.	HIV in combination therapy.
Enfuvirtide (Fuzeon)	**Fusion inhibitors.** Block HIV from entering CD4 T-cells	HIV in combination therapy.
Fostemsavir (Rukobia)	Binds gp120 on HIV to prevent CD4 cell entry.	HIV in combination therapy
Ibalizumab (Trogarzo)	**Post-attachment inhibitors.** Block CD4 receptors on the surface of T cells. HIV needs the CD4 receptor for cell entry.	HIV in combination therapy.
Lenacapavir (Sunlenca)	Interferes with HIV capsid	HIV in combination therapy
Combination HIV drugs	Approximately two dozen combination therapies are FDA approved and marketed (https://aidsinfo.nih.gov/understanding-hiv-aids/fact-sheets/21/58/fda-approved-hiv-medicines)	

Table 7.9 Pneumocystis carinii Agents

DRUG	MECHANISM	INDICATIONS	NOTES
Trimethoprim-sulfamethoxazole (e.g., Bactrim, Septra)	Inhibits folate synthesis pathway as demonstrated in Figure 7.13.	Oral dose form is drug of choice for PCP prophylaxis in immuno-suppressed patients. IV form is drug of choice for PCP infection.	See Table 7.5.
Pentamidine (Pentam)	Unknown.	Nebulized form used as alternative PCP prophylaxis. IV form is an alternative for PCP treatment.	Inhaled form frequently causes bronchospasm. Bronchodilators should be readily available.
Dapsone	Unknown	Alternative for PCP prophylaxis.	
Atovaquone (Mepron)	Unknown	Treatment for mild PCP in TMP-SMZ-resistant patients.	

VIRAL RESISTANCE	UNDESIRABLE EFFECTS	PHARMACOKINETICS	NOTES
	Rash, hepatotoxicity.	PO.	Contraindicated in renal function impaired patients.
	Dizziness, serious skin reactions.	PO.	
Mutations in reverse transcriptase (e.g., conversion of methionine at codon 184 to either isoleucine or valine.)	Peripheral neuropathy, pancreatitis, diarrhea, headache, insomnia, vomiting, nausea, rash, abdominal pain. Zidovudine-myelosuppression.	PO. Metabolized in liver, excreted in urine. Toxicity may be enhanced by renal or hepatic dysfunction.	Limited utility as single agent therapy because of viral resistance.
Mutations in protease sequence reduce affinity of protease inhibitors.	GI distress, headache, other neurologic symptoms (e.g., weakness, anorexia, parasthesias). **Indinavir** associated with increased risk of kidney stones.	PO. Metabolized P450 in liver. Reduce dose in patients with liver dysfunction. Poor CNS penetration.	Potentially serious drug interactions due P450 enzyme competition. See package insert.

Table 7.10 Antifungal Drugs

DRUG	ACTION	CLINICAL USE	UNDESIRABLE EFFECTS
Polyenes			
Amphotericin B (Fungizone, Abelcet, Ambisome)	Disrupts the plasma membrane of fungal cells. Amphotericin has greater affinity for ergosterol (component of fungal plasma membrane) than for cholesterol (mammalian).	DOC: Systemic fungal infections, fungal meningitis, and fungal urinary tract infections.	Poor therapeutic index (toxic at therapeutic dose). Fever/chills, nephrotoxicity (reduce risk by hydrating patient), hypokalemia, nausea, headache, thrombophlebitis, anemia.
Nystatin (e.g., Mycostatin)	" "	DOC: Intestinal *Candida* or thrush (oral *Candida*).	Few adverse effects reported when administered orally.
Azoles			
Fluconazole (Diflucan)	Inhibits fungal cytochrome P-450 enzymes. Damages plasma membrane by inhibiting sterol demethylation (an essential step in the synthesis of plasma membrane sterols).	Systemic histoplasmosis, blastomycosis, coccidiomycosis (including meningitis), or sporotrichosis. Opportunistic cryptococcosis, candidiasis. Candidal thrush, vaginitis, esophagitis.	Nausea, headache, rash, vomiting, diarrhea.
Itraconazole (Sporanex)	" "	Aspergillosis, histoplasmosis, blastomycosis, coccidiomycosis (not meningitis), sporotrichosis, paracoccidiomycosis. Local *Tinea* or Candidal infections. Better than ketoconozole for Sporothrix aspergillus.	Nausea, edema (rare), hepatitis. No gynecomastia or breast pain.
Clotrimazole (e.g., Lotrimin)	Mechanism unknown.	DOC: Candida, dermatophyte infections of the skin. Vaginal candidiasis.	
Miconazole (Monistat)	" "	Vaginal candidiasis, severe systemic fungal infections.	Phlebitis, pruritus, nausea, fever, rash, vomiting (if intravenous).
Posaconazole (Noxafil)	Blocks synthesis of ergosterol which is needed for fungal membranes.	Prevention of invasive Aspertillus or Candida. Oropharyngeal candidiasis resistant to itraconazole/ fluconazole.	Hypertension, hypotension, headache, rash, diarrhea, nausea, vomiting, hypokalemia.
Caspofungin (Cancidas)	Inhibits synthesis of beta (1,3)-D-glucan, which is needed for fungal cell walls.	Aspergillosis, candidemia, esophageal candidiasis.	Hypotension, diarrhea, vomiting.
Micafungin (Mycamine)	" "	Candidemia, esophageal candidiasis.	" "
Anidulafungin (Eraxis)	" "	" "	" "
Other			
Voriconazole Isavuconazonium	Blocks fungal 14 α – lanosterol demethylation	Aspergillosis, esophageal candidiasis, other fungal infections	Visual disturbances, rash, vomiting, hepatotoxicity,

PHARMACOKINETICS	NOTES
Slow IV for systemic infections, intrathecal for meningitis, bladder irrigation for cystitis. Metabolism poorly understood, no need to reduce dose with renal dysfunction.	Blood count, urinalysis, liver enzymes, blood urea-nitrogen, creatinine, & electrolytes should be checked before and during teatment. Liposome-encased amphotericin (Abelcet, Ambisome) produces less nephrotoxicity and infusion related toxicity.
PO. Negligable absorption, fecal excretion. Also topical.	
PO/IV. Long half-life. Excellent penetration of CSF, eye, urine. Hepatic metabolism. Excellent bioavailability.	No effects on testosterone synthesis. Circumvents need to use intrathecal amphotercin for *Coccidiomycosis* meningitis.
PO/IV. Requires acidic evironment for absorption. Accumulates over time, long half-life, poor CSF and urine penetration, hepatic metabolism.	No effect on testosterone, gluocorticoid synthesis.
Topical/PO (troches)/Vaginal cream and inserts.	
Vaginal suppositories/vaginal cream/topical/IV.	
PO/IV.	Strong CYP3A4 inhibitor.
IV (slow infusion, not bolus).	
" "	
" "	
IV for all indications except esophogeal candidiasis (PO).	

Antifungal Therapy

Fungi exist in a yeast form and a mold form. The yeast form reproduces by budding or spore formation and the mold form grows by extending hyphae (branches). A history of travel is particularly important when fungal infection is suspected because most types of fungi are endemic to specific regions.

Fungi are larger than bacteria and can usually be visualized microscopically without stain, particularly if nonfungal cells have been destroyed by 10% potassium hydroxide (KOH prep). Fungi are resistant to KOH because of their unique, rigid cell wall. Because human cells lack cell walls, antifungal therapy is directed primarily at destroying the fungal cell wall. Despite this apparent "selective" difference between human and fungal cells, antifungal agents are generally very toxic to human cells and should be used with caution.

Common Sites of Invasion:

- *Candida* most often infects the mouth (thrush) or the vagina, particularly in persons with impaired cell-mediated immunity. Thrush is generally treated with nystatin "swish and swallow," or clotrimazole troches and vaginitis is usually treated with miconazole. Systemic *Candida* infections occur in immunosuppressed patients and require intravenous amphotericin B.

- *Histoplasma capsulatum, Blastomyces dermatitidis, Coccidioides immitis and Aspergillus* infections generally present as pneumonia which may progress to systemic fungosis. Amphotericin B has traditionally been the drug of choice for such systemic infections. Fluconazole and itraconazole are newer drugs that rival amphotericin B with regard to efficacy for some systemic fungal infections. Amphotericin B requires intravenous infusion, but fluconazole and itraconazole are abailable in oral forms.

- *Cryptococcus neoformans* may also present as pneumonia, but more commonly presents as meningitis in immunosuppressed individuals. Fluconazole and flucytosine are the only antifungal agents that reach therapeutic concentrations in the brain. Of the two, fluconazole is more effective against *Cryptococcus*.

Anti-parasitic Therapy

Table 7.11 presents a partial list of agents used to treat parasites.

Widespread resistance to antimalarial drugs complicates therapy. The drug of choice for the treatment of malaria depends on the pattern of drug resistance in the region where the patient was infected. Individuals traveling to endemic regions are encouraged to take prophylactic antimalarial drugs.

Table 7.11 Antiparasitic Drugs

DRUG	MECHANISM	CLINICAL USE	UNDESIRABLE EFFECTS
Metronidazole (Flagyl) Tinidazole	Activated nitro intermediates bind DNA and inhibit anaerobe replication. Antiparasitic mechanism unknown.	Protozoans: *Entamoeba histolytica, Trichomonas, Giardia*. Anaerobes: *Bacteroides, Clostridium, Peptococcus*.	Seizures, ataxia, dizziness, nausea, anorexia, bloating, cramping. Disulfiram-like reaction.
Lindane (e.g., Kwell)	Induces seizures in ectoparasites.	Scabies (*Sarcoptes scabiei*): body, head, and pubic louse (*Pediculus capitis, P. corporis, Phthirus pubis*).	Topical administration may lead to seizures, CNS disturbances, risk of arrhythmias. Skin irritant.
Antihelminthic Drugs			
Mebendazole	Disrupts microtubules in worms.	DOC or pinworm. Also effective against roundworms.	Diarrhea, fever, GI pain. Highly contagious, family members should be treated.
Praziquantel	Increases cell membrane permeability causing loss of intracellular calcium. Results in paralysis of worms and release from host tissues.	Schistosome infections Single dose therapy is adequate.	Minimal side effects. Patients may feel like they have flu.
Thiabendazole	Unknown.	Strongyloidiasis, multiple parasite infection.	Flu symptoms, hepatotoxicity, anorexia, CNS disturbances.
Ivermectin (Stromectol)	Helminthic glutamate-gated channel antagonist causes worm paralysis.	Strongyloides, Onchocerca	Pruritis, rash, fever in onchocerciasis patients.
Antimalarial Drugs			
Chloroquine Hydroxy-chloroquine (Plaquenil)	4-aminoquinoline. Mechanism not clear. Wide resistance of unknown mechanism.	Prophylaxis or acute attacks. Erythrocytic forms of *P. falciparum*. Used in some auto-immune diseases (Lupus, Rheumatoid arthritis).	Dizziness, headache, irreversible retinal damage, impaired accommodation, bullseye retina, hemolysis in G6PD-deficient patients.
Quinine	Not Clear Increasing resistance in S.E. Asia.	Chloroquine resistant *P. falciparum*. Little effect on sporozoites or pre-erythrocytic stages.	Cinchonism, curare-like effects, shock. MOST TOXIC antimalarial (should only be used when other antimalarials fail).
Mefloquine	Not Clear. Structural analog of quinine.	Active against multidrug resistant malaria (including Chloroquine resistant *P. falciparum*.)	Well tolerated, benign sinus bradycardia Single dose cures multidrug resistant *P. falciparum* malaria.
Pyrimethamine	Inhibits folate synthesis by interfering with dihydrofolate reductase. Less resistance when used in combination with sulfonamides (Combination marketed as Fansidar®).	Malaria prophyaxis. Erythrocytic form of *P. falciparum*. Used in combination with sulfonamides or sulfones for acute attacks. Combined with Sulfadiazine for treating Toxoplasmosis.	Few, mild side effects.
Primaquine	Mechanism unclear. Likely to involve crosslinking of glutathione. Little resistance to drug by *P. vivax* (8-aminoquinoline).	Chloroquine resistant vivax malarias. More active against hepatic than erythrocytic forms of malaria.	Hemolysis in patients with G6PD-deficiency.

Chapter 8 **Anticancer Drugs**

Tumor cells are derived from normal cells in which proliferation is poorly controlled. Because tumor cells are similar to normal cells, it has been difficult to develop anticancer agents which selectively kill tumor cells without harming normal tissues.

Most anticancer agents act by inhibiting cell proliferation. Generally this is achieved by either damaging DNA or preventing DNA repair. Essentially, there are four ways in which most anticancer drugs inhibit proliferation:

- Crosslinking DNA. Prevents separation of DNA strands.
- Linking alkyl groups to DNA bases. Inhibits repair of DNA.
- Mimicking DNA bases, resulting in 1) incorporation of drug into DNA or RNA, where it prevents repair or terminates the chain or 2) negative feedback on enzymes that synthesize or recycle purines.
- Intercalating between base pairs of DNA, disrupting the triplicate codons or producing oxygen free radicals which damage DNA.

Hormonal anticancer drugs antagonize receptors, preventing endogenous growth-promoting hormones from binding (Table 8.5). Other hormonal agents are agonists at receptors that, when activated, inhibit tumor growth.

In caring for patients on chemotherapy, it is essential to evaluate the patient for dose-limiting side effects (some, such as permanent cardiomyopathy from Adriamycin, are initially asymptomatic), to know how to treat neutropenic fever, and to effectively manage nausea and vomiting.

Principles of Cancer Chemotherapy

• *The cell cycle*

Tumor cells are remarkably similar to noncancerous human cells. Thus, there are relatively few drug strategies for destroying tumor cells while sparing non-neoplastic cells. Newer agents selectively target cancer cells by using monoclonal antibody technology. Neoplastic and normal cells differ primarily with regard to the number of cells undergoing cell division, and most anticancer drugs act by killing cells that are dividing. The drugs accomplish this by interfering with DNA, RNA, or protein synthesis or by inhibiting the formation of microtubules in mitosis. Such agents are called cell cycle-specific agents because they exert their actions during distinct phases of the cell cycle (Fig. 8.1). In general, agents that interfere with DNA synthesis are S-phase specific; those that interfere with microtubules disrupt mitosis and are called M-phase specific.

DNA alkylating agents damage tumor cells regardless of whether the cell is actively dividing. Because of this property, these agents are called "cell cycle-nonspecific" drugs.

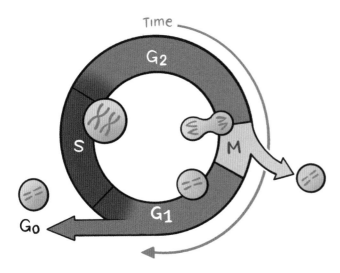

Figure 8.1 The cell cycle. *Cells pass through four stages of growth during each mitotic cycle. Cells that contain a double complement of DNA (G_2 cells) divide during mitosis (M phase). Following a "gap" (G_1 phase) cells may either differentiate and remain out of the cycle for a long period of time (G_0 period) or begin the process of DNA synthesis (S phase). Another gap (G_2) follows.*

• *Resistance and Recurrence*

If a tumor cell is to be killed by an anticancer drug, 1) the drug must reach the tumor cell, 2) the tumor cell must enter the phase of the cell cycle that is targeted by the drug, and 3) the cell must not be resistant to the drug.

Cancer cells become resistant to anticancer agents through a variety of mechanisms including 1) reduced uptake of drug into cell, 2) enhanced production of enzymes that repair damaged DNA, 3) production of chemically altered enzymes which are no longer recognized by drugs that inhibit unaltered enzymes, 4) reduced transformation of prodrugs (inactive precursors) into cytotoxic agents and 5) enhanced transformation of toxic agents into inactive metabolites.

Some tumors become resistant to several classes of antitumor agents, even if they have never been exposed to some of these agents. This is called multidrug resistance. Affected drugs include antibiotics, colchicine, the vinca alkaloids (vincristine & vinblastine) and epidophyllotoxins (VP-16). Cross-resistance among these agents is striking because they do not share a common mechanism of action.

Multidrug resistance is due to increased expression of an energy-dependent membrane glycoprotein "pump" which lowers the intracellular concentration of chemotherapeutic agents. The multidrug resistance gene is likely one of multiple genes that are induced to protect cells from toxic insults.

• *Toxicity of Anticancer Drugs*

Erythropoietic and leukopoietic cells, cells lining the gastrointestinal tract, and hair follicle cells are replaced at a much greater rate than most other non-cancerous cells in the normal human. Because of the rapid growth rate of these cells, they are susceptible to damage by anticancer drugs. Bone marrow suppression, mucositis, and alopecia are predictable side effects of most anticancer agents. In addition, many drugs cause toxicity that is unrelated to cell growth rate (Fig. 8.3).

• *Combination therapy*

Chemotherapeutic regimens often consist of several agents which have different mechanisms of action and minimize overlapping toxic effects. This affords multiple points of attack on the tumor cell while sparing normal organs from the toxicity produced by higher doses of a single drug. Most anticancer drugs cause bone marrow suppression. Bone marrow-sparing drugs (e.g., vincristine) are frequently included in combination regimens, if the tumor is sensitive.

Alkylating Agents

Alkylating agents were the first anticancer agents developed. They are chemically related to mustard gas which was used in World War I.

Alkylating agents are generally more effective against slow-growing tumors than other classes of antineoplastics because they are cell-cycle nonspecific. Relatively few cells in slow-growing tumors are mitotically active during a given course of chemotherapy. In contrast to most other agents, alkylator-induced damage to cancer cells accumulates even during quiescent portions of the cell cycle.

All alkylating agents are toxic to hematologic cells. Thus, myelosuppression is a predictable side effect. Alkylating agents may cause secondary tumors, even years after therapy. Important side effects are shown in Table 8.1 and Figure 8.3. Note which drugs are used to treat CNS tumors, not because they are better agents, but because they cross the blood brain barrier. Similarly, drugs that penetrate the blood-testis barrier are used to treat testicular cancer.

Antimetabolites

Antimetabolites are cell-cycle specific agents which prevent synthesis of nucleotides or inhibit enzymes by mimicking nucleotides.

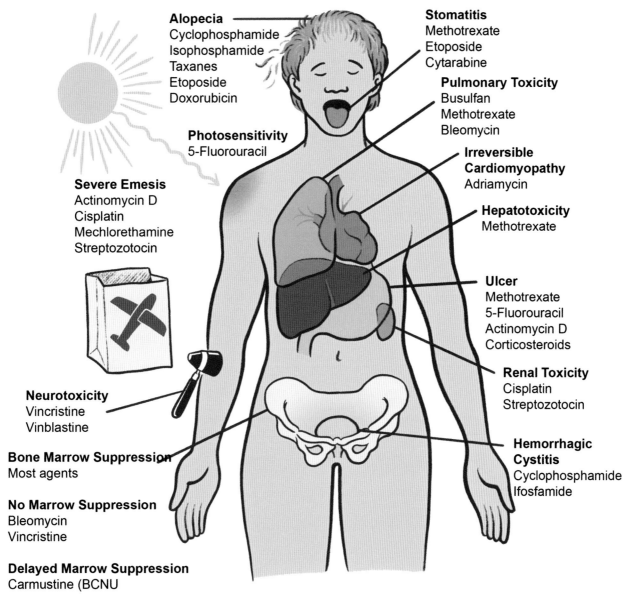

Figure 8.3 Notable side effects of chemotherapeutic agents.

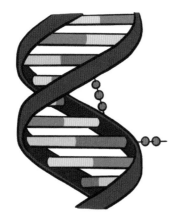

Figure 8.4 DNA alkylation. *Normally, DNA strands are joined by hydrogen bonds and other weak forces which allow separation during cell division. Bifunctional alkylating agents (alkylating group on both ends) covalently bind double stranded DNA together, preventing DNA transcription. Bifunctional alkylation is more toxic than single strand alkylation because it is less easily repaired.*

Methotrexate inhibits dihydrofolate reductase, an enzyme which reduces dihydrofolate (FH_2) to tetrahydrofolate (FH_4). Normally, the coenzyme FH_4 transfers a methyl group to dUMP, forming thymidylate, and is oxidized to FH_2 in the process. Methotrexate prevents recycling of this cofactor. Because thymidylate is necessary for DNA synthesis, methotrexate is toxic in the S-phase (synthesis).

Methotrexate toxicity to normal cells is reduced by supplying an alternative cofactor, leucovorin, or by bypassing the folate pathway by adding thymidine. Thymidine is converted directly to thymidylate by thymidine kinase. Administration of these agents after methotrexate is called leucovorin or thymidine "rescue." Leucovorin and thymidine do not "rescue" tumor cells from methotrexate because they do not reach adequate concentration in tumor cells.

Other antimetabolites used to treat cancer are either purine or pyrimidine analogs. In some cases,

Table 8.1 DNA Alkylating Agents

DNA Alkylating Agents: Nitrogen Mustards

Mechlorethamine **Chlorambucil** (Leukeran) **Melphalan** (Alkeran) **Cyclophosphamide** (Cytoxan) **Ifosfamide** (Ilex)	Alkylate DNA, which prevents DNA transcription, a necessary part of cell division. The actions on cancer cells are not cell cycle phase specific (drugs affect multiple phases of the cell cycle). The activities of alkylating agents are not specific to cancer cells, so they block cell division of most rapidly growing cells (e.g., blood cell precursors, hair cells, gut cells) which is the basis of common side effects (anemia, low platelets, impaired immune function, hair loss, nausea, gut toxicity). Cancers develop resistance by reducing cellular uptake of drugs or repairing DNA damage. Cyclophosphamide and ifosfamide are pro-drugs (inactive) that are metabolized to active forms in the liver. A toxic acrolein metabolite of cyclophosphamide can cause hemorrhagic cystitis, so Mesna, which binds the metabolite, is given to minimize bladder toxicity.

DNA Alkylating agents: Nitrosureas

Carmustine (BCNU) **Lomustine** (CCNU) **Streptozotocin** (Zanosar)	Similar to above.

DNA alkylating agents: Other chemical classes

Busulfan (Myleran) **Thiotepa** **Altretamine** (Hexalen) **Temozolomide** (Temodar) **Dacarbazine** (DTIC-Dome) **Procarbazine** (Matulane)	Similar to above. Cancer cells that are resistant to most alkylating agents are sometimes sensitive to altretamine (less cross resistance).

Table 8.2 Antimetabolites

Methotrexate	Blocks folate reduction by inhibiting dihydrofolate reductase. Dihydrofolate reductase (DHFR) reduces dihydrofolate to tetrahydrofolate, the coenzyme which is essential for the production of thymidylate. Drug is S-phase specific and also arrests some cells in G1, preventing them from entering S phase. Cancer cells develop resistance through decreased uptake, increased production of dihydrofolate reductase by gene amplification, altered forms of dihydrofolate, which are not recognized by methotrexate. In addition to usual toxicity of cytotoxic chemotherapy (decreased blood cell counts, nausea, hair loss), methotrexate can cause liver and kidney toxicity. When higher doses are administered, methotrexate serum levels are monitored to ensure that the patient is clearing the drug. While serum levels are above the threshold that can cause organ damage, leucovorin (formyl folate) is administered to "rescue" non-cancerous cells. Leucovorin restores reduced folate stores in non-cancerous cells. Methotrexate is also used to treat rheumatoid arthritis, psoriasis and other autoimmune disorders (due to cytotoxic effects on immune cells).
Purine Analogs	
Mercaptopurine (6-MP) **Thioguanine** (6-TG)	Mercaptopurine is metabolized to a ribose phosphate derivative (6MPRP) that mimics a negative feedback inhibitor to shut down purine production by cells. Thioguanine is metabolized to Thio-GTP or Thio-dGTP, which are incorporated into DNA where they block DNA repair or maintenance. Both kill cells during S-phase. Resistance occurs due to increased alkaline phosphatase (degrades 6MPRP), decreased sensitivity to feedback inhibition, or decreased HGPRT (the enzyme that metabolizes these drugs to toxic metabolites). Both kill cells during S-phase. Toxicity: decreased blood cell counts, nausea, hair loss, and liver damage. Doses are reduced if liver damage enzymes increase in blood.
Cladribine (Leustatin)	Metabolized intracellularly to 2-CdATP, which inhibits repair of single strand DNA. Incorporates into DNA of dividing cells. The metabolizing enzyme, deoxynucleotide deaminase, is reduced in non-cancerous monocytes and lymphocytes, which is why cancer cells are preferentially affected. Cladribine inhibits both DNA repair (non phase-specific) and DNA synthesis (S-phase). Resistance: High levels of deoxynucleotide deaminase (diverts 2-CdATP precursors into non-toxic pathway). Low levels of enzymes that synthesize 2-CdATP. Toxicity: decreased blood cell counts, nausea, hair loss.
Fludarabine (Fludara)	Metabolized to 2-fluoro-ara-ATP, which inhibits DNA polymerase, DNA primase and ribonucleotide reductase. Toxicity: decreased blood cell counts, nausea, hair loss.
Pyrimidine Analogs	
5-Fluoruracil **Capecitabine** (Xeloda)	Metabolized to fluoro-UMP which incorporates into RNA. Also metabolized to fluoro-dUMP which inhibits thymidylate synthetase. Floxuridine and capecitabine are prodrugs that are converted to fluorouracil in the body. All are S/G1 phase-specific. Drug resistance occurs due to decreased phosphorylation of prodrug to active form, increased intracellular catabolism, and increased or altered target enzyme. Toxicity: decreased blood cell counts, nausea, hair loss.
Cytarabine	Metabolized to ara-CTP, which is incorporated into DNA. Acts as a chain terminator and inhibits DNA polymerase. S-phase specific. Resistance and toxicity similar to above.
Gemcitabine (Gemzar)	Phosphorylated to dFdCDP and dFdCTP which inhibit ribonucleotide reductase. Also DNA strand terminator. S-phase specific. Resistance and toxicity similar to above.

the analogs are phosphorylated to nucleotides, then incorporated into DNA or RNA where they inhibit enzymes or result in faulty transcription or translation. Nucleotide analogs also inhibit essential enzymes such as thymidylate synthetase.

Miscellaneous Anticancer Agents

Antibiotic Anticancer Agents (Table 8.3) are drugs isolated from the fungal species *Streptomyces*. These drugs are classified together solely by their origin. They have different mechanisms, toxicities, pharmacokinetics and indications. Therefore, it is not useful to simply learn a prototype drug for this class. The most commonly used antibiotics are Adriamycin, Actinomycin D, mitomycin C and bleomycin.

Mitosis Inhibitors (Table 8.4) include agents that interfere with the microtubules that form during mitotic cell division. Microtubules are tubulin molecules that polymerize to form the spindles that segregate duplicated chromosomes. The vinca alkaloids depolymerize microtubules. In contrast, the taxanes stabilize the tubulin polymers so that they are unable to depolymerize, which is also necessary for cell division. Topoisomerase inhibitors block the enzyme that breaks and repairs DNA strands as chromosomes unwind during duplica

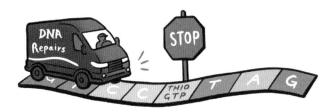

Figure 8.5 Antimetabolites such as thioguanine are incorporated into DNA where they inhibit repair or replication enzymes. Thioguanine is phosphorylated to thio-GTP which mimics GTP. The exact mechanism by which thio-GTP inhibits enzymes is unknown. The other purine and pyrimidine analogs work by similar mechanisms.

tion. The result is DNA strand breaks which that damage the genome and ultimately lead to cell death.

Kinase Inhibitors (Table 8.6) are typically designed to block the catalytic domain of tyrosine kinases. Tyrosine kinases are often involved in activating oncogenic signaling cascades that initiate or maintain cancer. The success of imatinib (Gleevec) for treating chronic myeloid leukemia led to intense and successful discovery efforts for other kinase targets. Rapid development of resistance to these drugs is often problematic.

Immuno-oncology Agents (Table 8.7) include monoclonal antibodies that induce cancer cell death through complement fixation (e.g., rituximab); block activity of

(continued on page 136)

Table 8.3 Antibiotic Anticancer agents

S phase specific	
Doxorubicin (Adriamycin) **Daunorubicin** **Idarubicin** **Epirubicin**	Anthracycline chemical structure. Intercalate into DNA, decrease DNA and RNA synthesis, cause DNA strand breaks via activity on topoisomerase II. Most notable side effect is irreversible cardiomyopathy. This risk is reduced by slow infusion and capping lifetime exposure. Also cause radiation recall, in which previously irradiated skin/tissue becomes inflamed. IV agents are used in combination with other agents for many types of cancer.
G2/M phase specific	
Bleomycin	Bithiazole rings intercalate into DNA strand. Drug oxidizes iron, which yields free radicals that damage DNA. Most notable side effect is pulmonary fibrosis. Test doses are given prior to administration because of risk of anaphylactic reactions. Used in combination therapies because it is less immunosuppressive than most cytotoxic agents. Indicated for testicular cancer, squamous cell head and neck cancer, and lymphomas.
Not phase specific	
Mitoxantrone (Novantrone)	Inhibits DNA and RNA synthesis, causes DNA strand breaks, inhibits topoisomerase II. IV agent used for acute non-lymphocytic leukemia.
Mitomycin C	This is an IV prodrug that is metabolized to an alkylating and crosslinking agent. IV drug used for adenocarcinoma of the stomach, colon, pancreatic and breast cancer along with squamous cell head and neck carcinoma.

Table 8.4 Mitosis Inhibitors and platinum containing agents

Vinca Alkyloids

Vincristine (Oncovin)	M-phase-specific agent binds tubulin and depolarizes microtubules. Used for leukemia, lymphoma, and some solid tumors. Toxicity includes neuropathy, constipation, jaw pain. Minimal bone marrow suppression.
Vinblastine	Similar mechanism as vincristine. Less neuropathy and more marrow suppression.
Vinorelbine	Similar mechanism. Used for non-small cell lung cancer, breast, ovarian, Hodgkins. Less neurotoxicity due to decreased affinity for nerve tubules.

Taxanes

Paclitaxel (Taxol)	M-phase specific. Stabilizes microtubules and prevents depolymerization that is necessary for mitosis. Used for metastatic ovarian carcinoma and breast cancer. Toxicity includes peripheral neuropathy, marrow suppression, myalgias, nausea, hypersensitivity reactions.
Albumin-bound Paclitaxel (Abraxane)	By formulating Paclitaxel with albumin, toxicity-inducing solvents in Paclitaxel were removed which improved the therapeutic index. Approved for metastatic breast cancer.
Docetaxel (Taxotere)	Similar to Paclitaxel. Less peripheral neuropathy.
Cabazitaxel (Jevtana)	Similar to Paclitaxel. Improved penetration of the blood brain barrier compared to Paclitaxel.

Topoisomerase Inhibitors

Etoposide (VePesid)	G2 Phase specific drug that interferes with topoisomerase, causing DNA strand breaks. Used for testicular and lung cancers. Causes marrow suppression, mucositis, nausea, and hypotension (associated with rapid infusion).
Topotecan (Hycamptin)	Interacts with topoisomerase I. Results in DNA strand breaks during replication. Used for lung and ovarian carcinoma. Causes marrow suppression.
Irinotecan (Camtosar)	Similar to topotecan. Used for metastatic colon carcinoma. Causes severe diarrhea in some patients.

Epothilones

Ixabepilone (Ixempra)	Promotes tubulin polymerization. IV drug used for metastatic breast cancer that has failed anthracyline and taxane therapy.

Platinum containing agents

Cisplatin (Platinol-AQ)	Mechanism unclear. Indicated for metastatic testicular tumors, ovarian tumors, advanced bladder cancer and some central nervous system tumors. Causes irreversible ototoxicity and nephrotoxicity. IV drug. Penetrates testes barrier and partially penetrates blood brain barrier.
Carboplatin (Paraplatin)	Similar to cisplatin. Fewer side effects that cisplatin and approximately equal in efficacy for lung cancer and ovarian cancer. Less effective than cisplatin for germ cell tumors, bladder cancer, and head and neck cancer.
Oxaliplatin (Eloxatin)	Similar to cisplatin. Small but significant improvement in efficacy for advanced colorectal cancer, where it is used in combination therapy.

Table 8.5 Miscellaneous Cancer Drugs

Vorinostat (Zolinza) **Belinostat** (Beleodaq) **Romidepsin** (Istodax)	**Histone Deacetylase (HDAC) inhibitors.** DNA is wrapped around histones and some cancers are caused or supported by genes that are abnormally expressed because of the interactions between histones and DNA. HDAC inhibitors prevent HDACs from deacetylating histones, which changes the expression level of many genes, some of which are integral to cancer growth.
Bortezomib (Velcade) **Carfilzomib** (Kyprolis) **Ixazomib** (Ninlaro)	**Proteosome inhibitors.** Proteins are degraded within cells by complexes of proteases in a structure called the proteasome. Proteins are targeted to the proteasome by the addition of a ubiquitin group. The balance between protein production and protein degradation contributes to cellular homeostasis. Certain cancer cells are particularly sensitive to disruption of this homeostasis by proteasome inhibitors. Administered by IV injection. Approved for lymphoma and multiple myeloma but not solid tumors.
Arsenic trioxide (Trisenox)	Induces degradation of the aberrant PML-retinoic acid receptor a fusion protein, which is likely involved in efficacy for acute promyelocytic leukemia. Also interferes with multiple other cellular signaling pathways and induces apoptosis in a number of cancer cell types *in vitro*.
Niraparib (Zejula) **Olaparib** (Lynparza) **Rucaparib** (Rubraca)	**PARP inhibitors.** PARP (Poly (ADP-ribose) polymerase plays a role in cellular growth and survival. Inhibition of PARP can reduce the ability of PARP to help cancer cells survive following DNA damage. Another gene/protein that helps cancer cells survive is called BRCA. In cancers, such as some breast cancers that have BRCA mutations, PARP is the only remaining mechanism to prevent cell death when there is DNA damage, so inhibiting PARP can lead to cancer cell death.
Venetoclax (Venclexta)	**BCL-2 inhibitors.** BCL-2 is an anti-apoptotic protein that can help cancer cells survive even when they have been treated with chemotherapy (BCL-2 causes resistance to some chemotherapies). Blocking BCL-2 enables the apoptotic cell death program to proceed. Used primarily in cancers that overexpress BCL-2, such as chronic lymphocytic leukemia (CLL).
Palbociclib (Ibrance) **Ribociclib** (Kisquali) **Abemaciclib** (Verzenio)	**CDK4/6 inhibitors.** Cyclin-dependent kinases 4 and 6 (CDK4/6) are active in the G1-S phase of the cell cycle, where they phosphorylate and inhibit members of the retinoblastoma protein family such as RB1. Phosphorylation of RB1 releases the transcription factor E2F, which activates transcription of genes that drive progression through G1/S phase. CDK4/6 inhibitors block cell cycle progression.
Ivosidenib (Tibsovo)	**Isocitrate dehydrogenase -1 (IDH1) inhibitors.** IDH1 is a cytoplasmic enzyme that decarboxylates isocitrate to yield a-ketoglutarate. Mutated IDH1 in cancers such as glioblastoma leads to abnormal production of 2-hydroxygluarate (2-HG). 2-HG inhibits histone and DNA demethylases, which alters gene expression and appears to drive cancers.
Vismodegib (Erivedge) **Sonidegib** (Odomzo) **Glasdegib** (Daurismo)	**Sonic hedgehog (shh) pathway inhibitor.** Blocks activity of the smoothened protein, which reduces shh activity. Indicated for shh pathway-driven cancers. Not effective for cancers that are driven by shh pathway activation that occurs downstream of the smoothened protein. May cause severe birth defects if used by pregnant women because the shh pathway is critical for embryo development.
Asparaginase (Erwinaze, Asparlas)	Hydrolyzes L-asparagine to aspartate. Lack of asparagines kills tumor cells that lack asparagine synthetase. Normal cells synthesize asparagine. Not phase specific.
Hydroxyurea	S-phase specific agent that inhibits ribonucleotide reductases. Blocks deoxyribonucleotide synthesis. Used for chronic granulocytic leukemia. Causes bone marrow suppression.
Mitotane	Isomer of DDT (a pesticide that is now banned). Specifically kills adrenocortical cells. Is used for palliative treatment of adrenocortical carcinoma. It is stored in fat and slowly released. Causes GI distress, lethargy, weakness, and dizziness.
Tretinoin (Vesanoid) **Isotretinoin** (Accutane)	Analog of retinoic acid (vitamin A) that induces maturation in acute promyelocytic leukemia cells and neuroblastoma. Toxicity includes the retinoic acid-syndrome (fever, dyspnea, pulmonary infiltrates and effusions, fluid retention), transient leukocytosis, pseudotumor cerebri.
Bexarotene (Targretin)	Selectively binds and activates the retinoid X receptor subtypes (RXRα, RXRβ, RXRY). These receptors act as transcription factors that regulate gene expression that encode proteins involved in cellular differentiation and proliferation. Used for refractory cutaneous T-cell lymphoma. Risk of severe birth defects.

Helpful Hint Regarding Drug Names:

-mab: Drugs with names ending in "mab" are **m**onoclonal **a**nti**b**odies. Monoclonal antibodies are large proteins that do not pass through the glomeruli in kidneys, so the proteins have a long serum half-life. For this reason, most monoclonal antibodies are administered intravenously about every 2-3 weeks. The downside of the long serum half-life is that it is difficult to stop the process if serious side effects occur.

-ib: Drugs with names that end in 'ib' are small molecule inh**ib**itors. Typically these are oral medications and many have been optimized by medicinal chemistry to require once a day dosing.

Table 8.6 Kinase and Growth Factor Receptor Inhibitors

Imatinib (Gleevec) **Dasatinib** (Sprycel) **Bosutinib** (Bosulif) **Ponatinib** (Iclusig) **Asciminib** (Scemblix)	**BCR-ABL tyrosine kinase inhibitors.** In certain cancers such as chronic myelogenous leukemia (CML), a translocation between chromosomes 9 and 22 creates a chimeric chromosome (Philadelphia chromosome, Ph+) with a novel fusion protein, called BCR-Abl at the junction. BCR-Abl is a tyrosine kinase that drives cancer. These agents inhibit the ABL kinase, and some are used for cancers in which upstream mutations increase the activity of ABL (e.g., PDGFRa mutations in gastrointestinal stromal tumors (GIST)). These kinase inhibitors inhibit kinases other than BCR-ABL to varying degrees, which influences both efficacy and side effects. Emergence of drug resistance is a problem for most kinase inhibitors. Very often this occurs by either a mutation in the drug binding site, which reduces the affinity of the drug for the target. Alternatively, some cancer cells use alternate signaling pathways ("pathway switching") to drive cell division and proliferation.
Gefitinib (Iressa) **Erlotinib** (Tarceva) **Lapatinib** (Tykerb) **Vandetanib** (Caprelsa) **Neratinib** (Nerlynx) **Osimertinib** (Tagrisso) **Dacomitinib** (Vizimpro) **Mobocertinib** (Exkivity)	**Epidermal growth factor (EGFR) inhibitors.** Bind to the tyrosine kinase extracellular domain of EGFR to block EGFR activity. EGFR normally functions to regulate epithelial tissue growth, development and homeostasis. EGFR mutations or amplifications drive lung, breast, brain and other cancers. EGFR inhibitors are most often prescribed for cancers with EGFR mutations or amplifications. These small molecule EGFR inhibitors (end in "ib") are oral and typically inhibit other kinases, which influences efficacy and side effects.
Cetuximab (Erbitux) **Panitumumab** (Vectibix) **Necitumumab** (Portrazza)	**Monoclonal antibodies that block EGFR.** The monoclonal antibodies (end in "-mab") are administered by IV, typically every 2-3 weeks, and are very specific to EGFR.
Sunitinib (Sutent) **Sorafenib** (Nexavar) **Axitinib** (Inlyta) **Cabozantinib** (Cometriq) **Ponatinib** (Iclusig) **Regorafenib** (Stivarga) **Vandetanib** (Capreisa) **Pazopanib** (Votrient) **Lenvatinib** (Lenvima) **Tirozanib** (Fotivda)	**Vascular endothelial growth factor (VEGF) receptor inhibitors.** These agents bind to the VEGF receptor and block the tyrosine kinase activity that is required for generating new blood vessels that are needed for cancer mass growth. All of these agents inhibit kinases other than VEGFR to varying degrees, which influences both efficacy and side effects. Like most small molecule drugs, these have serum half-lives of <24 hours, so they are typically administered as pills once a day.
Bevacizumab (Avastin, Mvasi) **Ramucirumab** (Cyramza)	**Monoclonal antibodies that block VEGFR.** Must be administered intravenously. Because antibodies have a very long half-life, these drugs are administered once every 2-3 weeks instead of daily. Because of the long half-life, it is necessary to stop these drugs about 4 weeks prior to a major surgery and about 4 weeks after surgery. These inhibitors are very specific to VEGFR, so have fewer side effects than the drugs above.
Ziv-aflibercept (Zaltrap)	**Recombinant humanized protein that antagonizes VEGF-A, VEGF-B and placental growth factor.** Risk of severe bleeding, gastrointestinal perforation and delayed wound healing due to on-target activity.

Table 8.6 Kinase and Growth Factor Receptor Inhibitors (continued)

Dabrafenib (Taflinlar) **Trametinib** (Mekinist) **Vemurafenib** (Zelboraf) **Ruxolitinib** (Jakafi) **Afatinib** (Gilotrif) **Ceritinib** (Zykadia) **Nintedanib** (Ofev) **Alectinib** (Alecensa) **Deucravacitinib** (Sotyktu) **Selpercatinib** (Retevmo) **Pemaglitinib** (Pemazyre) **Selumetinib** (Koselugo) **Encorafenib** (Braftovi) **Erdafitinib** (Balversa) **Pacritinib** (Vonjo) **Umbralisib** (Ukoniq) **Pexadartinib** (Turalio) **Infigratinib** (Truseltiq) **Tepotinib** (Tepmetko) **Capmatinib** (Tabrecta) **Entrectinib** (Rozlytrek) **Riprentinib** (Qinlock) **Futibanib** (Lytgobi) **Fedratinib** (Inrebic) **Pralsetinib** (Gavreto) **Vandetanib** (Capreisa) **Avapritinib** (Ayvakit)	**Multikinase inhibitors.** These agents inhibit multiple kinases, which influences both efficacy and side effects. Sometimes called "dirty" kinase inhibitors, these agents were typically intentionally designed to block multiple signaling pathways that are all important for cancer. Many of the signaling pathways are also important for noncancerous cells, so finding a therapeutic window in which the drugs kill cancer cells at doses that are well tolerated is challenging. Most other small molecule kinase inhibitors, but not the monoclonal antibodies, listed in Table 8.6 are also multikinase inhibitors. The spectrum of kinases that they inhibit and the affinity for each kinase influences the activity and toxicity of the drug.
Olaratumab (Lartruvo)	**Monoclonal antibody that blocks Platelet-derived growth factor receptor alpha (PDGFRα).** Elevated PDGFRa levels are associated with poor prognosis in sarcoma. In other cancers, PDGFRa mutations, fusions or amplifications are observed. Olartumab, with a standard chemotherapy agent, is used to treat sarcoma.

MAPK Pathway (RAS, RAF, MEK, ERK) Inhibitors

Vemurafenib (Zelboraf) ***Encorafenib** (Braftovi)	**BRAF inhibitors** used for melanoma and other tumors with BRAF V600 mutation. Selectively inhibits mutated form compared to nonmutated form, which provides cancer specificity. Side effects include rash, photosensitivity, alopecia, cutaneous squamous cell cancer, fatigue.
Trametinib (Mekinist)	**Mitogen-activated extracellular signal-regulated kinase (MEK) inhibitor.** Approved for use alone in selected patients with BRAF V600E or V600K mutation. Also approved for use in combination with a BRAF inhibitor for cancers that have BRAF mutations. Rash, diarrhea, bloody stools, edema.
***Binimetinib** (Mektovi) ***Cobimetinib** (Cotellic)	**MEK kinase inhibitors** used in combination with encorafenib for cancers with BRAF V600E or V600K mutation.

Table 8.6 Kinase and Growth Factor Receptor Inhibitors (continued)

PI3K/AKT/mTOR Pathway Inhibitors

Copanlisib (Aliqopa)	**Phosphoinositide 3-kinase alpha (PI3Kα) or delta (PI3Kδ) inhibitor.** Blocks B-cell receptor-mediated signaling and CXCR12-mediated malignant B cell chemotaxis. Also blocks NFkB signaling.
Alpelisib (Piqray)	Phosphoinisitide 3-kinase alpha (PI3Kα) inhibitor approved for hormone-positive, HER2-negative advanced breast cancer. Serious adverse reactions include hypersensitivity, severe cutaneous adverse reactions (SCARs), hyperglycemia, pneumonitis, diarrhea or colitis, and embryo-fetal toxicity.
Duvelisib (Copiktra)	**Phosphoinositide 3-kinase delta (PI3Kδ) or gamma (PI3Kγ) inhibitor.** Serious infections, diarrhea, colitis, skin reactions and pneumonitis occur with relatively high frequency. FDA risk evaluation and mitigation strategy is available to help doctors assess the risk:benefit ratio.
Everolimus (Afinitor) **Temsirolimus** (Torisel) **Sirolimus** (Rapamune)	**Mammalian target of rapamycin (mTOR) inhibitors.** The mTOR pathway is central to multiple cancer causing or cancer promoting receptor tyrosine kinase pathways. Used in renal cell carcinoma. Everolimus is also approved for tumors in patients with Tuberous Sclerosis, which involves overactivity of the mTOR pathway.

HER2 Inhibitors

Traztuzimab (Herceptin) **Pertuzumab** (Perjeta) **Margetuximab** (Margenza)	Monoclonal antibodies that bind to the extracellular domain of human epidermal growth factor receptor 2 (HER2) protein. Approved for breast cancers that overexpress HER2.
Lapatinib (Tykerb) **Neratinib** (Nerlynx) **Dacomitinib** (Vizimpro) **Tucanitib** (Tukysa)	Small molecule inhibitors of the tyrosine kinase domain of HER2. Approved for HER2-positive breast cancer.

Other Tyrosine Kinase Inhibitors

Ibrutinib (Imbruvica) **Acalabrutinib** (Calquence) **Pirtobrutinib** (Jaypirca) **Zanubrutinib** (Brukinsa)	**Bruton's tyrosine kinase (BTK) inhibitor.** BTK is necessary for B cell development and BTK inhibitors are used for B cell malignancies. Because BTK inhibitors affect both normal and cancerous B cells, BTK inhibitors are also used to treat chronic graft-versus-host disease. Toxicity: Diarrhea, thrombocytopenia, neutropenia, edema,fatigue, dizziness, headache, anxiety, rash.
Midostaurin (Rydapt) **Gilteritinib** (Xospata) **Crenolanib**	**FLT-3 kinase Inhibitor.** FLT3 tyrosine kinase regulates proliferation and survival of hematopoietic stem and progenitor cells. FLT3 is mutated in about 1/3 of acute myelogenous leukemia (AML) patients. FLT3 inhibitors reduce peripheral blasts (AML progenitor cells) but have little effect on blasts in the bone marrow, so remissions occur rarely in response to this class of drugs.
Crizotinib (Xalkori) **Brigatinib** (Alunbrig) **Lorlatinib** (Lorbrena) **Alectinib** (Alecensa)	**ALK tyrosine kinase inhibitors.** ALK tyrosine kinase plays a role in brain development and is also expressed in small intestine and testes. Fusions that involve ALK and other genes cause non-small-cell lung cancer and anaplastic large cell lymphomas and ALK inhibitors are used in patients with these mutations. Toxicity: Edema, numbness, headache, dizziness, and irregular heartbeat.
Larotrectinib (Vitrakvi) **Entrectinib** (Rozlytrek)	**Oral selective tropomyosin receptor kinase (TRK) inhibitor.** Approved for use in solid tumors with neurotrophic TRK (NTRK)-fusion proteins. NTRKs are receptors for neurotrophic growth factors, which induce NTRK autophosphorylation and activation of downstream MAPK pathway. Larotrectinib was the first drug to be approved across all cancers provided that they have a specific genetic mutation, in this case the NTRK fusion. Toxicity: fatigue, nausea, cough, constipation, diarrhea, elevated liver enzymes (AST, ALT).

Table 8.7 Immuno-oncology Agents

Checkpoint Inhibitors (monoclonal antibodies)

Ipilimumab (Yervoy) **Tremelimumab** (Imjudo)	**CTLA-4 Inhibitors.** Monoclonal antibody that blocks the cytotoxic T lymphocyte antigen 4 (CTLA-4). CTLA-4 suppresses T cell activation, including tumor infiltrating lymphocytes (T cells that have potential to recognize and kill cancer cells). Ipilimumab therefore augments T-cell activation and proliferation. It is used for melanoma. Toxicities include immune mediated inflammation of various tissues and organs.
Pembrolizumab (Keytruda) **Nivolumab** (Opdivo) **Cemiplimab** (Libtayo)	**PD-1 inhibitors.** Monoclonal antibodies that block programmed death ligand 1 (PD-L1) from binding to PD-1 on activated T cells. PDL-1 binding to PD-1 normally causes the activated T cell to become docile or die. PD-1 inhibitors therefore augment T-cell activation and proliferation. Toxicities include immune mediated inflammation of various tissues and organs.
Avelumab (Bavencio) **Atezolizumab** (Tecentriq) **Durvalumab** (Imfinzi) **Dostaslimab** (Jempesli)	**PD-L1 inhibitors.** Monoclonal antibody binds to PD-L1 (as opposed to its receptor, PD-1).

Antibody-Drug Conjugates

Brentuximab vedotin (Adcetris)	Monoclonal antibody that delivers monomethyl auristatin E (MMAE) to cancer cells that express **CD30** (e.g., Hodgkins Lymphoma). The MMAE enters the cells and disrupts microtubules, causing cell death.
Ado-trastusumab emtansine (Kadcyla)	Monoclonal antibody that delivers emtansine to cancer cells that express **HER2** (e.g., breast cancer). Shown to provide benefit to HER2-positive breast cancer patients, including those who previously failed Herceptin.
Moxetumomab pasudotox-tdfk (Lumoxiti)	Fc fragment of an anti-CD22 monoclonal antibody that delivers the *Pseudomonas* exotoxin-A to cells that express CD22, such as hairy cell leukemia cells. Toxicity: capillary leak syndrome, hemolytic uremic syndrome, renal toxicity and electrolyte imbalance. Because **CD22** is expressed on normal B cells, the B cell population (which makes antibodies) is diminished as a side effect.
Gemtuzumab Ozogamicin (Mylotarg)	Monoclonal antibody that delivers the cytotoxic agent calicheamicin to cells that express **CD33**, such as acute myelogenous leukemia (AML).
Inotuzumab Ozogamicin (Besponsa)	Monoclonal antibody that delivers the cytotoxic agent calicheamicin to cells that express **CD22**, such as B-cell precursor acute lymphoblastic leukemia (pre-B-ALL). Toxicity: liver toxicity including veno-occlusive disease (VOD).
Polatuzumab vedotin (Polivy)	Binds **CD79** and is used for diffuse large B-cell lymphoma.
Enfortumab vedotin (Padcev)	Binds **Nectin-4** and is used for urothelial cancer.
Trastuzumab deruxtecan (Enhertu)	Binds **HER2** and is used for breast cancer.
Sacituzumab govitecan (Trodelvy)	Binds **Trop-2** and is used for metastatic triple negative breast cancer.
Lonastuximab tesirine (Zynlonta)	Binds **CD19** and is used for Large B-cell lymphoma.
Tisotumab vedotin	Binds **tissue factor** and is used for cervical cancer.
Mirvetuxumab soavtansine (Elahere)	Binds **Frα** and is used for ovarian cancer.

Table 8.7 Immuno-oncology Agents (Continued)

Monoclonal Antibodies (Monoclonal antibody receptor tyrosine kinase (RTK) inhibitors are in Table 8.6)

Rituximab (Rituxan) **Ofatumumab** (Arzerra) **Ibritumomab** (Zevalin) **Obinutuzumab** (Gazyva) **Ocrelizumab** (Ocrevus) **Epcoritamab** (Epkinly) **Ublituximab** (Briumvi)	Monoclonal antibodies that block **CD20**, which is expressed on B-cell leukemias and lymphomas. Postulated to induce complement-dependent cytotoxicity. CD20 is also present on normal B cells, but not normal B cell precursors. Therefore, patients normal B cell may be damaged by these antibodies causing transient immunodeficiency, but are later replaced.
Tafasitamab (Monjuvi)	Monoclonal antibody that blocks **CD19**, which is expressed on B cell leukemias and lymphomas. Used to treat large cell leukemia. Toxicities include neutropenia, thrombocytopenia, elevated glucose, hypocalcemia, and many others.
Alemtuzumab (Campath)	Recombinant humanized MAB that binds to **CD52**, an antigen on B and T lymphocytes. Approved for B-cell chronic lymphocytic leukemia.
Mogamulizumab-kpkc (Poteligeo)	Recombinant humanized MAB that binds to **CCR4**, which is the receptor for five chemokines (CCL2, CCL4, CCL5, CCL17, and CCL22). These chemokines normally regulate trafficking of white blood cells, making them important for the function of the immune system. Used for subtypes of cutaneous T-cell lymphoma.
Daratumumab (Darzalex) **Isatuximab** (Sarclisa)	Recombinant humanized MAB that binds to CD38, a cell surface protein that is highly expressed in multiple myeloma and is also expressed on normal white blood cells.
Dinutuximab (Unituxin)	Chimeric human-mouse anti-glycolipid disialoganglioside (anti-**GD2**) antibody used to treat neuroblastoma.

Bispecific or Multispecific Antibodies

Blinatumomab (Blincyto)	Bispecific or multispecific antibodies typically bind to two or more targets to cause cancer cell death. For example, **blinatumomab binds to CD19** on lymphoblastic leukemia **and to CD3** on T cells. Blincyto connects the T cell to the cancer cell and through activation of CD3, causes T cells to kill cancer cells. Non-cancerous cells that express the target are often also killed, in this case B cells that express CD19.
Amivantamab (Rybrevant)	Binds to **EGFR and c-MET**, both on cancer cells. Blocks dual signal pathways and is approved for non-small cell lung cancer.
Tebentafusp (Kimmtrak)	Binds to **gp100** on cancer cells and **CD3** on T cells. Approved for metastatic uveal melanoma.
Mosunetuzumab (Lunsumio)	Binds to **CD20** on cancer cells and **CD3** on T cells. Approved for refractory follicular lymphoma.
Teclistamab (Tecvayli)	Binds to **BCMA** on cancer cells and **CD3** on T cells. Approved for multiple myeloma.

Other Immuno-oncology Agents

Thalidomide (Thalidomid) **Lenalidomide** (Revlimid) **Pomalidomide** (Pomalyst)	Thalidomide was originally removed from the market after use as an anti-emetic in pregnant women led to limb defects in newborn babies. With intensive safety precautions to avoid birth defects, it was approved for multiple myeloma patients. Thalidomide binds to and blocks the protein cereblon, which leads to immunomodulation, which is likely responsible for anti-cancer activity. Lenalidomide is used for anemia, multiple myeloma, myelodysplastic syndrome in patients with 5q chromosome deletion. Pomalidomide is used for multiple myeloma.
Interferon	Enhance activity of cytotoxic-T, natural killer cells and macrophages. Inhibit proliferation of tumor cells. Used for hairy cell leukemia, AIDS-related Kaposi's sarcoma. Other uses under investigation.

(continued from page 128)

oncogenic proteins (e.g., cetuximab); or bind to the proteins that are necessary for vascularization and growth of solid tumors (e.g., bevacizumab). Some monoclonal antibody classes (anti CTLA-4, anti PD-1, anti PDL-1) were designed to "take the brakes off" the immune system. For certain tumors, typically with many mutations, tumor infiltrating lymphocytes have cancer killing potential, but are negatively regulated by the CTLA-4 and PD-1/PDL-1 pathwaysare negatively regulated... [incomplete sentence?]. Blocking these targets with therapeutic antibodies induces an anti-cancer immune response in a subset of patients.

Other Anticancer Agents

The vinca alkaloids, vincristine, vinblastine, and vinorelbine inhibit tumor growth by destroying microtubules which are essential for cell structure and mitosis. They differ in that vinblastine and vinorelbine "blasts" bone marrow while vincristine spares marrow. Vincristine however, causes peripheral neuropathy which is manifested by decreased reflexes, foot drop, weak fingers and decreased autonomic function.

Etoposide (VP-16) is a synthetic derivative of epipodophyllotoxins. It appears to act by inhibiting topoisomerase, causing DNA strand breaks. VP-16 is used to treat small and nonsmall lung cancer, testicular cancer, and non-Hodgkins lymphoma.

Mitotane is remarkable simply because it preferentially accumulates in adrenocortical cells. Although treatment is not curative, mitotane is used to decrease symptoms caused by adrenal carcinoma.

Hormonal Anticancer Agents

Most anticancer hormones act as agonists that inhibit tumor cell growth or as antagonists that compete with endogenous growth promoting hormones. Adrenocorticosteroids inhibit multiple cell processes necessary for division. Leuprolide and Goserelin act at the pituitary to reduce LH and FSH secretion. LH and FSH promote growth of prostate cancer cells. Estramustine relies on the estrogen moeity simply to target the other half of the drug, which is an alkylating agent, into estrogen receptor-positive cells.

Table 8.8 Hormonal Anticancer Agents

DRUG	REMARKS
Hormones	
Estrogen	Estrogen receptor agonist which counteracts endogenous testosterone (testosterone enhances tumor growth) in patients with prostate cancer.
Progestin	Progesterone receptor agonist used to treat endometrial carcinoma, metastatic renal carcinoma and breast cancer. Mechanism of action unclear.
Tamoxifen	Estrogen receptor antagonist. Prevents endogenous estrogens from stimulating tumor growth. Used to treat estrogen receptor-positive breast cancer in postmenopausal women. Increased risk of uterine cancer observed in women treated with tamoxifen.
Aromatase Inhibitor	Non-steroidal aromatase inhibitor selectively reduces circulating estradiol levels for the treatment of advanced breast cancer (anastrazole and letrozole).
Androgen	Testosterone receptor agonists active against some breast and renal cancers.
Flutamide	Testosterone receptor antagonist which augments late effects of leuprolide and inhibits transient side effects caused by initial leuprolide-induced LH and FSH secretion.
Abiraterone (Zytiga)	Prodrug is converted in vivo to abiraterone, which inhibits androgen biosynthesis. The drug blocks CYP17, which is expressed in testicular, adrenal and prostatic tumor tissues and is required for androgen biosynthesis. Abiraterone is used with prednisone for treatment of castration-resistant (androgen antagonists no longer work) metastatic prostate cancer.
Adrenocortico-steroid	Inhibit DNA and protein synthesis as well as mitosis. Used for acute lymphocytic leukemia, chronic lymphocytic leukemia, acute myelogenous leukemia, multiple myeloma, breast cancer, lymphoma.
Leuprolide, Goserelin	Analog of gonadotropin releasing hormone (GNRH). Desensitizes GNRH receptors in pituitary, causing decreased release of gonadotropin. Results in decreased sex hormone release and is used for advanced prostate cancer. Initially stimulates transient release of sex hormones (LH and FSH).
Estramustine (EmCyt)	Estrogen agonist linked to alkylating agent. Drug uptake is enhanced in estrogen receptor-positive cells, causing selective accumulation of alkylating agent in tumor cells. Used for prostate carcinoma.

Leukemias and lymphomas are derived from immune cells, so it makes sense that agents which regulate division of immune cells might also affect tumor cell growth. Interferons are protein products that were isolated from immune cells and are now produced using recombinant DNA technology. Interferons induce a number of gene products in cells that are interferon receptor-positive. In addition, they stimulate activity of certain immune cells, some of which may act against tumor cells.

Hematopoietic Agents

The agents listed in Table 8.9 differ from all the other drugs in this chapter. These are not chemicals, isolated from plants or synthesized in a lab. They are glycoproteins produced by cultured mammalian cells, into which the gene for erythropoietin, G-CSF or GM-CSF has been introduced. Because they are identical or nearly identical to endogenous hematopoetic agents, there are relatively few side effects.

These agents are extremely expensive to develop and produce. The investment has led to exciting new therapeutic interventions, however, which were impossible with conventional drug development techniques. Recombinant DNA technology is now being applied to numerous medical problems, particularly those due to paucity of an endogenous substance (e.g., insulin in diabetes mellitus).

The agents listed below reduce the need for blood transfusions in patients with chronic anemia, reduce the incidence of life-threatening infections in patients with low neutrophil counts, and improve the success of autologous bone marrow transplantation in cancer patients.

Table 8.9 Hematopoetic Agents

DRUG	DESCRIPTION
Epoetin alpha (e.g., Epogen)	Epoetin alpha is recombinant human erythropoetin. Erythropoetin, which is synthesized in the kidney in response to hypoxia or anemia, stimulates erythropoiesis. Epoetin alpha is indicated for anemia in patients with chronic renal failure, because these patients are unable to synthesize erythropoetin to correct the anemia. Additional uses include correcting zidovudine (AZT)-induced anemia in HIV-infected patients and chemotherapy-induced anemia in cancer patients. Several weeks of therapy are required before the hematocrit levels rise, therefore, this drug cannot replace transfusions for the acute treatment of severe anemia. Epoetin alpha should not be used in patients with uncontrolled hypertension because the elevation in hematocrit may exacerbate hypertension.
Filgrastim (G-CSF) (Neupogen)	Filgrastim is human recombinant granulocyte colony stimulating factor (G-CSF), which induces synthesis of neutrophils from progenitor cells. Indicated for replenishment of neutrophils in cancer patients treated with myelosuppressive anticancer agents. The goal is to prevent neutropenia, which is associated with life-threatening bacterial infections. In the past, neutropenia-associated infection was the dose-limiting toxicity of many chemotherapeutic agents. Now, filgrastim permits the development of chemotherapy protocols that include higher doses of myelosuppressive drugs. This will likely result in higher treatment success, but will also result in the development of toxicities that were previously rarely seen, because the toxicities are produced only at high doses. Filgrastim should not be used within 24 hours of the administration of anticancer drugs because the effect of cytotoxic agents on rapidly dividing myeloid cells is not clear. The theoretical concern that filgrastim might act as a growth factor for malignancies has not been substantiated clinically. Filgrastim is indicated for the treatment of severe cyclic neutropenia and severe chronic neutropenia. The most frequent undesirable effect is medullary bone pain, likely due to rapid cell proliferation within the marrow.
Sargramostim (GM-CSF) (Leukine)	Sargramostim is human recombinant granulocyte-macrophage colony stimulating factor (GM-CSF). It stimulates the proliferation of all lines of blood cells. It induces maturation of granulocytes and macrophages, but not erythrocytes or megakaryocytes. Sargramostim also activates mature granulocytes and macrophages. The principle indication is to accelerate bone marrow replenishment following autologous bone marrow transplantation. It is under investigation for the treatment of several other myelosuppresive disorders. As with G-CSF, the possibility that GM-CSF might act as a growth factor for some types of cancer has not been ruled out.
Oprelvekin (Interleukin II, Neumega)	Oprelvekin is a recombinant growth factor that stimulates platelet production. It is indicated for maintaining platelet counts following chemotherapy. Clinical trials show limited efficacy. Toxicity includes fluid retention, tachycardia and other cardiovascular reactions.

Chapter 9 Anti-inflammatory and Immunomodulating Agents

Drugs presented in this chapter modulate inflammation or other immune responses. Most of these agents influence other cellular functions as well, and are discussed in other chapters. The reason for the multitude of actions is that these agents generally interfere with processes that are vital to multiple biochemical pathways.

A beautiful example of a drug with such pleiotropic effects is aspirin. Aspirin reduces inflammation, lowers the temperature of febrile patients, relieves moderate pain and prevents blood clots. The biochemical mechanism of these actions is inhibition of the enzyme, cyclooxygenase. Cyclooxygenase catalyzes the synthesis of potent chemical messengers called prostaglandins, which regulate inflammation, body temperature, analgesia, platelet aggregation and numerous other processes.

In producing inflammation, the role of prostaglandins is to "call in" the immune system. Local tissue infiltration by immune cells and the release of chemical mediators by such cells cause the symptoms of inflammation (heat, redness, tenderness). Thus, a second mechanism for reducing inflammation involves inhibiting immune functions. In the past, this was accomplished using nonspecific immunosuppressants such as corticosteroids (presented in Chapter 10). Recent advances in immunology fueled the development of more selective agents, capable of inhibiting or stimulating specific immune pathways.

Such agents permit exciting new therapeutic approaches to organ transplantation, hyper- and hypo-immune diseases and cancer.

A third mechanism for treating inflammation involves antagonizing the effects of chemicals released by immune cells. Histamine, released by mast cells and basophils in response to antigens, causes bronchial constriction and inflammation by binding to histamine receptors on bronchial cells. Antihistamines are antagonists which compete with histamine for these receptors.

Like prostaglandins, histamine regulates numerous processes, including acid and pepsin secretion in the stomach, heart rate and vasodilation. Histamine antagonists which prevent acid and pepsin secretion are clinically used to treat peptic ulcer disease (Table 6.1).

Prostaglandin Inhibitors

Until a few years ago, there were two ways to pharmacologically reduce inflammation. One approach was corticosteroids. The other was the chemically-diverse agents known as "non-steroidal anti-inflammatory drugs" or NSAIDs (Tables 9.1, 9.2 and 9.3).

NSAIDs were used before their mechanism of action was understood. Ample evidence indicates that NSAIDs act by preventing prostaglandin synthesis. They will likely be referred to as prostaglandin synthesis inhibitors in the future.

Prostaglandins are a family of potent arachidonic acid metabolites, which modulate some components of inflammation, body temperature, pain transmission, platelet aggregation and a host of other actions. They are not stored by cells, but are synthesized and released on demand. Prostaglandins are rapidly degraded, so their half-life is in the range of seconds to minutes.

Aspirin and other NSAIDs inhibit cyclooxygenase, a critical enzyme in prostaglandin synthesis. Because this enzyme plays a role in the synthesis of all members of the prostaglandin family, NSAIDs tend to inhibit all prostaglandin functions (Tables 9.1 and 9.2).

Acetaminophen (e.g., Tylenol®) parallels aspirin with regard to its antipyretic (fever reducing) and analgesic effects, yet it lacks anti-inflammatory and antithrombotic actions. Because it produces less GI irritation than aspirin, it was introduced as an aspirin

Aspirin
(Acetylsalicylic Acid)

Acetaminophen

substitute. Soon, acetaminophen was used in place of aspirin for fevers, analgesia and *inflammation*, even though acetaminophen is a poor anti-inflammatory drug. This illustrates the hazard of equating similar drugs with one another rather than learning important differences.

The use of aspirin-like drugs for arthritis illustrates one problem associated with selective drug distribution. Many drugs fail to penetrate into joint spaces. High doses of aspirin or other non-steroidal anti-inflammatory agents (NSAIDS) are required to achieve therapeutic levels in the joint space. Of course toxicity to tissues other than joints is more likely at high drug concentrations. Gastrointestinal irritation and ulceration are likely to develop when high-dose NSAIDs are employed unless anti-ulcer drugs are concurrently administered to prevent gastroduodenal mucosa damage.

Antiarthritic Agents

Joint inflammation and tissue damage characterize arthritis. Antiarthritic agents include prostaglandin inhibitors (Table 9.2), corticosteroids (Table 10.6), other immunosuppressants (Table 9.3), and other antiarthritic agents (Table 9.3). The efficacy of antiarthritic agents depends on the type of arthritis being treated (Table 9.5).

The most important characteristics of antiarthritis drugs are 1) ability to reduce inflammation, 2) ability to reach therapeutic concentrations in joint capsules without reaching toxic levels in serum. Drugs in Tables 9.2 and 9.3 are the primary antiarthritic agents.

Nonsteroidal anti-inflammatory agents are used most frequently for arthritis. The major toxicity of these drugs, when used at doses large enough to penetrate joint capsules, is GI irritation and breakdown. Celecoxib (Celebrex®) and (now discontinued) rofecoxib (Vioxx®) are selective cyclooxygenase-2 inhibitors. Because they do not inhibit cyclooxygenase-1, there are fewer GI side effects at doses that are effective for arthritis. Antacids, H2 blockers, or prostaglandin analogs are prescribed to prevent or reverse NSAID damage to GI mucosa (Table 6.1).

Antigout Agents

Sodium urate crystallizes in joints, inciting an inflammatory reaction called tophaceous gout. Aspirin-like drugs may relieve the symptoms of gout, but therapy is more often directed at lowering uric acid levels. Uric acid is a product of purine metabolism. Strategies for reducing uric acid levels include inhibiting xanthine oxidase, the enzyme responsible of uric acid synthesis, and preventing uric acid reabsorption from the urine. Antigout drugs are described in Table 9.4.

Immunomodulating Agents

Immunosuppressants help prevent rejection of transplanted organs and bone marrow, prevent erythroblastosis fetalis (destruction of fetal blood cells by maternal antibody-mediated immunity) and may reverse autoimmune diseases such as aplastic anemia. They work by a variety of mechanisms (Table 9.6).

Some immunosuppressants are not drugs, but are instead antibodies that are produced by non-human animals and are directed at human immune cells. **Immunostimulants**, primarily investigational at this time, may be employed in the future for the treatment of AIDS, other immunosuppressed states, cancer, and viral diseases. Interferons and interleukins are peptides released by immune cells in the body (Table 9.6).

Table 9.1 Acetaminophen and Nonsteroidal Anti-inflammatory Agents (NSAIDS)

Acetaminophen (Tylenol)	Weak inhibitor of prostaglandin synthesis. Analgesic and antipyretic (fever) properties similar to NSAIDs below, but the anti-inflammatory effects are much weaker. Indicated for mild to moderate pain, but not used for disorders that are primarily inflammatory (e.g., rheumatoid arthritis). Compared to NSAIDs, has much lower risk of GI upset, GI bleeding, or platelet dysfunction. Overdose may cause hepatic necrosis leading to coma or death.
NSAIDS	
Acetylsalicylic acid (aspirin)	Inhibits cyclooxygenase (COX), an enzyme required for the synthesis of prostaglandins (prostaglandins mediate inflammation, fever & pain). "inflammation and pyrogen-induced fever." pain caused by injury or inflammation. Prevents platelet aggregation. Uses: Symptomatic relief of minor pain, inflammation, fever, or rheumatoid arthritis. Reduction of stroke risk. Toxicity: GI upset & bleeding, allergic reactions. Increased risk of Reye's Syndrome in children. Tinnitis. Increases risk of bleeding when used with anticoagulants.
Comments in right column below list the ways that each drug differs from aspirin	
Colecoxib	Cox-2 inhibitor
Diclofenac	No significant differences
Diflunisal (Dolobid)	Less likely to cause GI bleeding and tinnitis, but may cause acute interstitial nephritis.
Fenoprofen (Nalfon)	More potent than aspirin. Fewer GI side effects, more genitourinary side effects (pain on urination, hematuria, nephropathy).
Ibuprofen (Advil, Motrin)	Better tolerated than aspirin by most patients. Reduces diuretic effects of furosemide and may reduce effectiveness of several antihypertensive agents.
Indomethacin (Indocin)	Contraindicated in patients with GI lesions. May worsen pre-existing depression, epilepsy or Parkinson's disease. Most likely to be nephrotoxic. Also indicated to close patent ductus arteriosus in newborns.
Ketoprofen	Administered IV. More effective than aspirin for controlling pain.
Ketorolac (Ioradol)	The only parenteral nonsteroldal antl-Inflammatory for pain relief. Initial clinical trials indicate that it is equal to narcotic analgesics for controlling postoperative pain. IV/IM/PO dosing forms available for short-term pain management. No other indications.
Meclofenamate (Meclomen)	Induces diarrhea in 10–35% of patients.
Naproxen (Naprosyn)	Better tolerated than aspirin.
Olsalazine (Dipentum)	Pro-drug is metabolized to 5-aminosalicylic acid. It is retained in the colon, making it effective against ulcerative colitis.
Piroxicam (Feldene)	In addition to inhibiting prostaglandin synthesis, piroxicam prevents neutrophil aggregation and release of lysosomal enzymes.
Sulindac (Clinoril)	Fewer GI side effects than aspirin.
Mafenemic acid (Ponstel)	Prescription oral NSAID used for more severe pain, particularly menstrual pain.

Table 9.2 Rheumatoid Arthritis (RA) Drugs

NSAIDS (see table 9.1)	Block cyclooxygenase (COX1 and COX2), which reduces prostaglandin synthesis. Prostaglandins are essential for inflammation. Because prostaglandins are also important for platelet stickiness, gastrointestinal bleeding can be a side effect. Proton pump inhibitors (e.g., omeprazole/Prilosec) can be used to counteract GI toxicity.
COX2 inhibitors Celecoxib (Celebrex)	Inhibit COX2, which reduces inflammation, but does not inhibit COX1, which is responsible for many of the GI side effects. For patients who chronically need NSAID relief from inflammation, this class of drugs offers an alternative with fewer side effects.
Corticosteroids **Prednisone** **Methylprednisolone** (Medrol) **Triamcinolone**	Corticosteroids reduce inflammation by suppressing the function of immune cells. Because the immune system is suppressed, risk of infection increases. Other side effects include osteoporosis, hypertension, weight gain, increased blood sugar, avascular bone necrosis, and cataracts. Osteoporosis risk can be reduced by Vitamin D and calcium supplements along with bisphosphonates (e.g., alendronate). Corticosteroids can be given orally or by IV and some (e.g., triamcinolone) are injected directly into the joint. Intraarticular administration improves symptoms only at the injected joint and has the benefit of reduced systemic toxicity.

Disease Modifying Anti-rheumatic Drugs (DMARDs)
The following drugs slow joint damage in contrast to drugs above

Methotrexate (Rheumatrex, Trexall)	Methotrexate, given at lower doses than used for cancer treatment, reduces inflammation and joint damage by suppressing proliferation of immune cells through the inhibition of dihydrofolate reductase (enzyme necessary for folic acid metabolism). Considered first line DMARD since it is often effective and well tolerated for prolonged periods of time. Onset of relief occurs in 4-6 weeks. Rare but serious toxicities: hepatic cirrhosis, interstitial pneumonitis, severe myelosuppression. Common side effects: headache, fatigue, liver injury. Side effects can be reduced by co-administration of leucovorin.
Hydroxychloroquine	This antimalarial drug acts through an unknown mechanism to reduce the pain and inflammation of joint disease in RA. Typically used with sulfasalazine and methotrexate in a combination called triple therapy. Response usually seen in 2-4 months and drug is considered to have failed if no response is seen by 6 months. Rare but serious eye toxicities are observed, so it is important to evaluate for retinopathies before starting drug.
Sulfasalazine (Azulfidine)	Mechanism unknown. Usually used with methotrexate and hydroxychloroquine. Sulfa drug hypersensitivity occurs in some patients. GI distress can be reduced by using enteric coated tablets. Screen for deficiency of glucose-6-phosphate dehydrogenase (G6PD) before administering to avoid hemolysis in G6PD deficient patients.
Leflunomide (Arava)	Mechanism unknown. Alternative to methotrexate. Monitor liver enzymes. Avoid administration to pregnant women.
Etanercept (Enbrel) **Infliximab** (Remicade) **Adalimumab** (Humira) **Certolizumab pegol** (Cimzia) **Golimumab** (Simponi)	**Tumor necrosis factor (TNF) inhibitors.** All block TNF. Etanercept is a fusion protein made from the TNF receptor and the Fc domain of an immunoglobulin. The others are monoclonal antibodies. All are administered by injection. Onset of symptom relief is 2-4 weeks. Toxicities: increased risk of infection including opportunistic infections (e.g., tuberculosis, fungal infections), reactivation of Hepatitis B. Risk of some cancers may increase.
Abatacept (Orencia)	**T-cell costimulatory blockers.** T cells require stimulation through CD3 and co-stimulation through CD28 or other costimulatory receptors to become fully activated. Since activated T cells contribute to RA joint damage, these drugs bind to CD28 in a way that blocks CD28-mediated T-cell co-stimulation
Rituximab (Rituxan)	**B-cell depletion.** Rituxan is an antibody that binds to CD20, which coats B cells. Antibody binding leads to depletion of B cells, which contribute to RA. It is used in some patients who failed TNF inhibitors. Toxicities: Infusion reactions (immune system recognizes antibody as "foreign"), risk of Infections, Hepatitis B reactivation.
Tocilizumab (Actemra) **Sarilumab** (Kevzara)	**Interleukin-6 (IL-6) inhibitors.** IL-6 is a pro-inflammatory cytokine produced by immune cells. Monoclonal antibodies that bind IL-6 reduce RA joint damage. Toxicity: Infection risk, thrombocytopenia, liver toxicity, neutropenia, elevated lipids.
Anakinra (Kineret)	**Interleukin-1 (IL-1) inhibitors.** IL-1 is a pro-inflammatory cytokine produced by immune cells. Monoclonal antibodies that bind IL-1 reduce RA joint damage. Toxicity: Injection site reactions, increased infection risk.
Tofacitinib (Xeljanz) **Baricitinib** (Olumiant) **Upadacatinib** (Rinvoq)	**Janus kinase (JAK) inhibitor.** The JAK/STAT pathway induces transcription of genes that are involved in inflammation. JAK inhibitors are used in RA patients that have failed TNF inhibitors. Toxicity: Sometimes fatal infections (TB, bacterial, fungal, viral), potential increased risk of cancer.

Table 9.3 Gout and Uric Acid Lowering Drugs

NSAIDS **Colchicine** **Corticosteroids**	**Pain and inflammation relievers.** NSAIDS (ibuprofen, indomethacine), low dose oral colchicine (often in combination with NSAIDS) and corticosteroids (prednisone, methylprednisolone) are used for symptom relief.
Allopurinol (Zyloprim) **Febuxostat** (Uloric)	**Xanthine oxidase inhibitors.** Decrease uric acid levels by inhibiting xanthine oxidase, the enzyme that converts hypoxanthine to xanthine and xanthine to uric acid. Used for gout and to foster elimination of uric acid released from leukemia cells during initial chemotherapy for leukemia cancer patients.
Probenecid	**Renal absorption of uric acid inhibitor.** Competes with uric acid for renal reabsorption at the proximal convoluted tubule. Important to maintain good fluid intake sufficient to achieve 2-3 liters of urine output per day. Administer prophylactic dose of colchicine for initial 3-6 months because probenecid can induce gout flares.
Lesinurad (Zurampic)	**Uric acid transporter-1 (URAT1) and organic anion transporter-4 (OAT4) inhibitors.** Reduces the activity of these two apical transporters to block reabsorption of uric acid by the kidneys. Usually used in combination with allopurinol or febuxostat. Important to assess renal function during treatment as renal failure may occur.
Pegloticase (Krystexxa)	**Recombinant modified urate oxidase (uricase) enzyme.** Catalyzes the oxidation of uric acid to allantoin, which is readily excreted by the kidneys. Drug is administered subcutaneously and is pegylated to increase duration of action. Used in patients who have failed more conventional drugs. Toxicity: Anaphylaxis and infusion reactions occur because the immune system recognizes the protein as "foreign".

Table 9.4 Psoriasis Drugs

Traditional medications	Psoriasis has traditionally been treated with a variety of topical medicines (corticosteroids, retinoids, coal tar, tacrolimus, pimecrolimus). Oral medications have been used as well, though these carry risks of systemic toxicity. Oral treatments include Vitamin D, methotrexate, cyclosporine, retinoids, and apremalast (phosphodiesterase type 4 (PDE4) inhibitor). Newer therapies that are directed at the cytokines (IL23 and IL17) that drive the autoimmune cascade in psoriasis are described below.
Risankizumab **Guselkumab** **Tildrakizumab** (Ilumya)	**IL-23 Inhibitors.** Activated myeloid dendritic cells release IL-23, IL-17 and other cytokines to activate T-cells and other immune cells in a pro-inflammatory cascade that leads to keratinocyte proliferation, angiogenesis, and movement of immune cells into psoriatic lesions. These monoclonal antibodies are delivered subcutaneously at multi-week intervals.
Secukinumab (Cosentyx) **Ixekizumab** (Taltz) **Brodalumab** (Siliq) **Tumor necrosis factor (TNF) inhibitors.** See Table 9.2	**IL-17α Inhibitors.** See above – similar to IL-23 inhibitors.

Table 9.5 Multiple Sclerosis (MS) Drugs

Injectable medications

Interferon beta-1 (Avonex, Betaseron, Extavia, Plegridy, Rebif)	Identical to human interferon beta. Mechanism of action unknown. First line therapy in relapsing remitting MS. Clinical trials showed fewer exacerbations, reduced risk of disability progression and reduction of MS lesions in the brain. Toxicity: Depression, suicide, psychotic disorders, hepatic injury, heart failure, seizures.
Glatiramer (Copaxone)	Induces and activates drug-specific suppressor T-cells that downregulate autoimmune response against myelin (the lipid sheath that coats neurons and is damaged in MS) antigens. First line therapy in relapsing remitting MS. Toxicity: allergic reactions to drug, chest pain after 1 month of treatment.
Ofatumumab (Kesimpta)	Blocks **CD20**, which causes depletion of B cells. Ofatumumab is also used for chronic lymphocytic leukemia (CLL) because CLL cells express CD20.
Peginterferon beta-1a (Plegridy)	Immunosuppressant that reduces inflammation of the myelin sheath of nerve cells. Approved for relapsing MS.

Oral medications – For patients who prioritize convenience

Teriflunomide (Aubagio)	**Pyramidine synthesis inhibitor.** Mechanism for relieving MS is unclear. Has been used safely in combination with interferon beta and glatiramer. Toxicity: Severe hepatotoxicity (uncommon), alopecia, diarrhea, nausea, paresthesia.
Fingolimod (Gilenya) **Ozanimod** (Zeposia) **Ponesimod** (Ponvory) **Siponimod** (Mayzent)	**Blocks lymphocyte egress from lymph nodes via sphingosine 1-phosphate (S1P) receptor.** Results in fewer lymphocytes in circulation, hence less autoimmune attack on myelin sheaths in MS patients. Toxicity: Severe infection risk, arrhythmias, progressive multifocal leukoencephalopathy, macular edema, encephalopathy, respiratory decline, liver injury. Ozanimod and Siponimod are selective for fewer sub-types of ZS1p receptors. Ponesimod has a longer half-life than Fingolimod.
Dimethyl fumarate (Tecfidera) **Monomethyl fumarate** (Bafiertam) **Diroximel fumarate** (Vumerity)	**Reduces CD8 T cells.** Exact mechanism unclear. Seems to be better tolerated than Fingolimod and may be more effective than Teriflunomide based on clinical experience. Toxicity: anaphylaxis, progressive multifocal leukoencephalopathy, lymphopenia, flushing.

Drugs administered by continuous infusion – For patients with more active disease and those that prioritize efficacy over convenience and safety

Alemtuzumab (Campath)	**Monoclonal antibody against CD-52.** Because of safety concerns, usually reserved for patients who have not responded well to two or more disease modifying drugs.
Ocrelizumab (Ocrevus) **Ublituximab** (Briumvi)	**Monoclonal antibody against CD-20**
Natalizumab (Tysabri)	**Monoclonal antibody against α4-integrin.** Preferred by some physicians because of clinical trial data showing superiority over interferon beta-1 for reducing relapses.
Mitoxantrone (Novantrone)	**Cancer chemotherapy drug that interferes with topoisomerase II.** Topo II inhibition impairs proliferation of B-cells, T-cells, and macrophages; impairs antigen presentation; and blocks cytokine secretion.

Table 9.6 Other Immunosuppressants and Immunostimulants

DRUG	MECHANISM/ACTIONS	INDICATIONS	UNDESIRABLE EFFECTS
Immunosuppressants			
Cyclosporine (Sandimmune, Neoral)	Inhibits T-Cell-mediated immunity by 1) ↓ production of interleukin-II by activated T-helper cells, 2) ↓ the number of interleukin receptors on cytotoxic-T cells, 3) allowing proliferation of T-suppressor cells.	Agent of choice for preventing and treating transplanted organ rejection. Graft versus host disease in bone marrow transplant.	Nephrotoxicity (presentation is similar to kidney rejection!), thromboembolism, neurotoxicity, seizures, reversible hepatotoxicity, hypertension.
Tacrolimus (Prograf)	Suppresses T-lymphocyte activity. Mechanism not clear.	Transplant organ rejection, graft vs. host.	Nephrotoxicity, neurotoxicity.
Azathioprine (Imuran)	Converted to 6-mercaptopurine ribose phosphate which inhibits purine synthesis. Because DNA & RNA synthesis requires proteins, all proliferating cells are inhibited (B-cells, T-cells, nonimmune cells).	Prevention of organ transplant rejection.	GI distress, bone marrow depression, infections, mild leukopenia and thrombocytopenia.
Mizoribine (Bredinin)	Inhibits guanine nucleotide synthesis	Renal transplant	Fewer undesirable effects than azathioprine.
Cyclo-phosphamide (e.g., Cytoxan)	PRODRUG is converted by liver to an alkylating agent which crosslinks DNA. Proliferation of B-cells is inhibited more than T-cells. May also attack immunocompetent lymphocytes to inhibit established immune responses.	Drug of choice for Wegener's granulomatosis. Also used for severe rheumatoid arthritis & autoimmune blood disorders.	Alopecia, GI distress, hemorrhagic cystitis of the bladder, bone marrow depression.
Lymphocyte immune-, anti-thymocyte-globulin (Atgam)	Horse IgG antibodies which selectively suppress T-lymphocytes (cell-mediated immunity) and humoral immunity.	Prevention of organ transplant rejection, aplastic anemia.	Fever, chills, leukopenia, thrombocytopenia, skin reactions. Less often: arthralgia, chest or back pain, dyspnea, vomiting, nausea, headache, night sweats.
RhoD Immune Globulin (e.g., RhoGAM)	Human immune globulin which prevents sensitization of Rho negative recipients to Rho(D) positive blood. Theoretically binds to Rho(D) antigens, masking them from antigen-sensitive immune cells.	In Rho(D) negative mother carrying Rho(D) positive fetus or planning abortion. Goal: prevent erythroblastosis fetalis in future infants.	Generally well tolerated.

Corticosteroids (Tables 10.5 & 10.6), Nonsteroidal Anti-inflammatory Agents (Tables 9.1 & 9.2), Methotrexate (Table 8.2).
Basiliximab, Daclizumab, Muromonab-CD3, and Mycophenolate Mofetil are also used to prevent graft rejection in transplant settings.

DRUG	MECHANISM/ACTIONS	INDICATIONS	UNDESIRABLE EFFECTS
Immunostimulating Agents			
Levamisole (Ergamisol)	Stimulates cell-mediated immunity.	Colon cancer (Duke's stage C), in conjunction with fluorouracil.	Dermatitis, agranulocytosis, GI distress, malaise.
Interferons	Enhance activity of cytotoxic-T, natural killer cells, and macrophages. Inhibit proliferation of tumor cells and suppress graft-versus-host disease.	Hairy-cell leukemia, genital warts, Kaposi's sarcoma, chronic myelocytic leukemia.	Fever, headache, myalgias.

PHARMACOKINETICS	DRUG INTERACTIONS	NOTES
Oral most common, but absorption is erratic. IV for acute organ rejection. Metabolized by liver. No dose adjustment necessary with renal dysfunction.	Synergistic nephrotoxicity with amphotericin B, aminoglycosides & trimethoprim. Drugs which induce liver metabolizing enzymes may shorten half-life of cyclosporine.	Cyclosporine does not inhibit antibody-mediated (B-cell) immunity. Therefore, transplant patients are not at significant risk for microbial infections during cyclosporin therapy. Other drugs (corticosteroids), however, may suppress the patient's antimicrobial defenses.
PO/IV. Absorption is erratic.	Many drugs alter plasma concentration. Follow levels.	Similar efficacy to cyclosporin. Occasionally effective in patients that have failed a cyclosporin trial. Vice versa.
PO/IV. Prodrug is metabolized to 6-mercaptopurine (6MP). 6MP is converted to 6-thiouric acid by xanthine oxidase. Renal excretion.	ALLOPURINOL inhibits xanthene oxidase activity, thus increasing serum azathioprine levels.	6-Mercaptopurine is an anticancer agent (Table 8.2).
PO	Immune suppressants	
PO. Must be hydroxylated by the P450 system to the active form of the drug.		Encourage patients taking cyclophosphamide to drink plenty of fluids and void often to prevent hemorrhagic cystitis.
IV. Must have filter in IV line to prevent insoluble material from entering the bloodstream.		Anaphylaxis occurs in <1% of patients. An airway and appropriate drugs should be at the bedside during the course of therapy. Often administered with steroids to reduce risk of anaphylaxis.
IM.		Contraindicated in Rho(D) positive patients or in Rho(D) negative patients who have already developed anti-Rho(D) antibodies. are unknown.
		INVESTIGATIONAL. May suppress immune system in some cases. Clinical efficacy for treatment of various cancers is being determined.

Table 9.7 Antihistamines

DRUG	MECHANISM	CLINICAL INDICATIONS	UNDESIRABLE EFFECTS
Release Inhibitor			
Cromolyn Sodium (Nasalcrom)	Inhibits release of histamine from mast cells.	Prophylaxis of bronchial asthma & seasonal allergic conjunctivitis.	Well tolerated. Local irritation, headache, unpleasant taste.
Ethanolamines			
Diphenhydramine (Benadryl) **Clemastine** (Tavist) **Carbinoxamine**	H1 Receptor Antagonist	Type I allergies (allergic rhinitis & conjunctivitis, simple urticaria, pruritis, angioedema). To induce sleep.	Sedative: VARIABLE Anticholinergic: HIGH GI upset: LOW
Alkylamines			
Chlorpheniramine **Brompheniramine** (Dimetane) **Dexchlorpheniramine** (Polaramine)	" "	" "	Sedative: LOW-MODERATE Anticholinergic: MODERATE GI upset: LOW
Phenothiazine:			
Promethazine (Phenergan)	" "	" "	Sedative: HIGH Anticholinergic: HIGH
Piperidines[1] & Piperazines[2]			
[1]**Cyproheptadine** **Desloratadine** (Clarinex) [2]**Hydroxyzine** (Atarax) [2]**Meclizine** (Antivert)	" "	Type I allergies. Hydroxyzine is also used for treatment of anxiety and pruritis. Meclizine is used for motion sickness and vertigo.	Sedative: LOW-MODERATE Anticholinergic: MODERATE
Nonsedating antihistamines			
Loratadine (Claritin) **Fexofenadine** (Allegra) **Cetirizine** (Zyrtec) **Azelastine** (Astelin)	" "	Seasonal allergic rhinitis.	Little or no sedation.
H2 Receptor Antagonists – Described in detail in Table 6.1			
Cimetidine (Tagamet) **Ranitidine** (Zantac) **Famotidine** (Pepcid) **Nizatidine** (Axid) **Levocetirizine** (Xyzal)	H2 Receptor Antagonist	Duodenal/gastric ulcer, hypersecretion of acid.	Well tolerated. Diarrhea, dizziness, headache.

Table 9.8 Histamine Actions

RECEPTOR	ORGAN	ACTIONS	BIOCHEMICAL MESSENGERS
H1	Lung	Constrict bronchial smooth muscle	Stimulate cyclic GMP
H1	Adrenal Medulla	Stimulate catecholamine release	" "
H1	Veins	Constrict	" "
H1	Capillaries	Increase permeability	" "
H1	Gastrointestinal Muscle	Contract	" "
H2	Heart	Increase rate	Stimulate cyclic AMP
H2	Stomach	Increase HCl and pepsin secretion	" "
H1 & H2	Capillaries & arterioles	Dilate	Stimulate phosphatidyl inositol and ↑ Na^+ and Ca^{++} permeability of membranes.
H1 & H2	Heart	Increase contractility	" "
H3	Histamine-releasing cells	Inhibit histamine release	

CONTRAINDICATIONS	PHARMACOKINETICS	DRUG INTERACTIONS	NOTES
	Nasal spray, oral. Poorly absorbed, not metabolized.		Requires 4–6 doses per day to prevent reaction.
Anticholinergic activity may aggravate bronchial asthma, urinary retention, glaucoma.	Duration: 4–6 hrs. Metabolized in liver, excreted in kidney.		Slow onset prevents use in anaphylaxis.
" "	Duration: 4–25 hrs.		
" "	Duration: 4–26 hrs.		
" "			
Concurrent use of erythromycin (macrolide), ketoconazole, itraconazole.	Don't cross blood brain barrier. Rapid, extensive metabolism, high plasma protein binding.	Potentially fatal arrhythmias with erythromycin, ketoconazole, itraconazole.	
Use cimetidine with caution in >50 year olds w/kidney or liver failure.	Little plasma protein binding, little metabolism.	Cimetidine ↑ levels of many drugs (e.g., oral anticoagulants, theophylline, caffeine, phenytoin, phenobarbital, benzodiazepines, propranolol) by inhibiting liver P450 enzymes.	

Antihistamines

Ragweed pollen, bee stings and other antigens elicit immune responses ranging from mild wheezing to potentially-fatal anaphylactic shock in sensitive individuals. Histamine, a chemical produced in many human tissues, mediates many of these responses. Mast cells and basophils release histamine in response to a variety of antigens.

Following release, histamine binds to either H1 or H2 histamine receptors causing a variety of effects (listed in Table 9.8). In addition to allergens, several other substances cause histamine release, including radiodiagnostic dyes, some antibiotics, kinins (chemicals released by immune cells) and some venoms. Several synthetic histamine agonists are available for laboratory studies of histamine functions, but there are virtually no clinical indications for histamine receptor agonists.

Histamine antagonists, on the other hand, are among the most widely used drugs. The term "antihistamines" generally refers to drugs which block H1 histamine receptors. These agents prevent bronchial smooth muscle contraction and inhibit histamine-induced vasodilation and increased capillary permeability. Therefore, H1 antihistamines are particularly useful for treating allergies.

H2 antagonists inhibit acid and pepsin secretion in the gastrointestinal tract and are used to treat peptic ulcer disease (Table 6.1).

Both H1 and H2 histamine receptor antagonists act by competing with histamine that has been released. A second strategy for reducing histamine-induced symptoms involves preventing histamine release from mast cells and basophils. Inhibitors of histamine release are available for *prophylaxis* against allergy and asthma symptoms (Table 9.7).

Chapter 10 **Endocrine System**

Endocrine glands release endogenous chemicals, called hormones, into the bloodstream to regulate the function of target tissues. This chapter addresses endocrine functions which are modified by clinically useful drugs.

The pituitary gland regulates virtually every endocrine gland and is often called the "master gland." It is divided anatomically and functionally into an anterior and a posterior lobe.

Anterior Pituitary Hormones

The hypothalamus secretes releasing and inhibitory substances into the anterior pituitary vasculature, thereby regulating anterior pituitary function. Pituitary secretions are also controlled by feedback control via circulating hormones. Endocrine systems influenced by the anterior pituitary are:

- **Sex Hormones:** The pituitary glycoprotein hormones, luteinizing hormone (LH) and follicle stimulating hormone (FSH), control sex steroid synthesis, spermatogenesis, follicular development and menstruation. The hypothalamic peptide, gonadotropin-releasing hormone (GnRH), stimulates the release of both LH and FSH from the pituitary. Circulating sex steroids inhibit the release of LH and FSH; inhibin, a peptide synthesized in the gonads, selectively inhibits FSH. Synthetic GnRH agonists initially stimulate LH and FSH secretion, then desensitize the pituitary, resulting in decreased LH and FSH secretion. **Nafarelin acetate** (Synarel®), **leuprolide** (Lupron®) and **goserelin**

(Zoladex®) are indicated for endometriosis. **Histrelin acetate** (Supprelin®), **nafarulin acetate** (Synarel®) and **leuprolide** (Lupron Depot) are indicated for precocious puberty. **Gonadorelin** (Lutrepulse®) is indicated for primary hypothalamic amenorrhea.

- **Adrenal steroids:** Corticotropin-releasing factor (CRF), a hypothalamic releasing factor, stimulates release of corticotropin (ACTH) from the pituitary gland. ACTH stimulates the adrenal gland to produce corticosteroid hormones (Tables 10.5–10.7). Cleavage of the precursor pro-opiomelanocortin (POMC) yields ACTH and another glycoprotein, β-lipoprotein (Fig. 3.5). β-lipoprotein further converts to the endogenous opioid peptide endorphin. Likewise, melanocyte stimulating hormone (MSH) results from the cleavage of ACTH.

- **Thyroid hormones:** Thyroid stimulating hormone (TSH), released by the pituitary gland, facilitates synthesis and release of thyroxine (T_4) and triiodothyronine (T_3). TSH is a glycoprotein composed of two chains, designated α and β. The α chain of TSH is identical to the α chain of FSH, LH and human chorionic gonadotropin (hCG). TSH release is stimulated by thyrotropin-releasing factor (TRH), a hypothalamic peptide. Serum T3 and T4 are feedback inhibitors of TSH synthesis. They also act as TRH antagonists in the pituitary.

- **Growth Hormone:** Pituitary growth hormone (GH) is released by growing children in discrete pulses, late in the sleep cycle. Hypothalamic growth hormone-releasing factor (GRF) stimulates GH and the hormone somatostatin (SRIF) inhibits it. Somatostatin is released from the hypothalamus, the gastrointestinal tract and the pancreas. It acts as a neurotransmitter. Inadequate secretion of growth hormone results in dwarfism. Recombinant human growth hormone is available by prescription (Somatrem®, Somatropin®). Synthetic GH contains the 191 amino acid sequence of pituitary-derived GH. Both endogenous and synthetic GH induce skeletal and organ growth and promote anabolic metabolism. **Octreotide** (Sandostatin®) is an analog of somatostatin, which inhibits growth hormone. It is used clinically to treat acromegaly.

- **Prolactin:** Prolactin is an anterior pituitary hormone which induces milk secretion from the breasts of lactating women. Nipple stimulation promotes prolactin release and dopamine inhibits prolactin release. **Cabergoline** (Dostinex®) is indicated for hyperprolactinemia

Posterior Pituitary Hormones

The posterior pituitary stores and releases two octapeptides, vasopressin and oxytocin, which are synthesized in the supraoptic and paraventricular nuclei of the hypothalamus. Both polypeptides are carried to hypothalamic nerve endings in the posterior pituitary by the transport protein, neurophysin.

- **Vasopressin:** Arginine vasopressin peptide (AVP, antidiuretic hormone) promotes reabsorption of water in the distal tubules and collecting ducts of the kidney and vasoconstricts blood vessels. It is released from pituitary nerve terminals in response to hypotension. Vasopressin deficiency results in **diabetes insipidus**, a disorder which is remarkable for polyuria (excessive urine production) and polydipsia (excessive thirst). **Vasopressin** (Pitressin®), **lypressin** (Diapid®) and **desmopressin** (DDAVP, Stimate®) are synthetic analogs of arginine vasopressin used for treatment of diabetes insipidus (intranasal or intravenous). They act rapidly and their antidiuretic actions persist for 8–20 hours.

Desmopressin is indicated for acute epistaxis (intranasal) and GI hemorrhage (intravenous). It is also used to maintain hemostasis during surgical procedures in patients with hemophilia A and Von Willebrand's disease. The mechanism of platelet function enhancement is unknown.

- **Oxytocin:** The posterior pituitary also releases oxytocin, an octapeptide that differs from vasopressin by two amino acids. Oxytocin induces contractions in the gravid uterus and promotes milk ejaculation from the post-partum breast. Uterine relaxants and contractants are discussed in Table 10.3.

Other Hormones

The pituitary does not control the endocrine pancreas or the parathyroid glands. The endocrine pancreas produces insulin, which regulates serum glucose levels. Pancreatic hormones are discussed on pages 153–155.

Parathyroid hormone (PTH), vitamin D and calcitonin work in synchrony to regulate calcium homeostasis (not

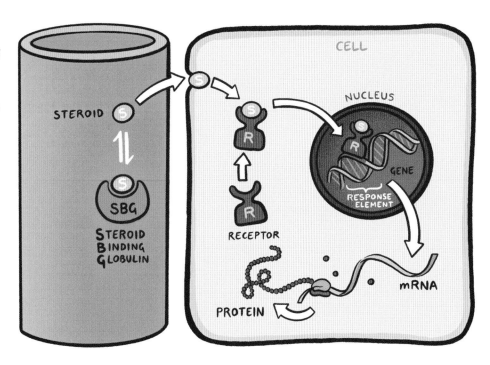

Figure 10.1 Mechanism of Steroid hormone action. Steroid hormones (S) circulate bound to steroid binding globulins (SBG). The free steroid penetrates plasma membranes and bind to cytoplasmic receptors (R). The steroid-receptor complex enters the nucleus, and binds to specific response element DNA sequences, regulating transcription of target genes.

presented in tables). **PTH** is an 84 amino acid chain secreted by the parathyroid glands in response to low serum calcium. PTH induces bone resorption, which liberates calcium into the bloodstream. These actions are dependent on adequate serum concentrations of 1,25-dihydroxy cholecalciferol (a derivative of vitamin D). Bone resorption is counterregulated by **calcitonin**, which inhibits osteoclasts (the cells which degrade bone).

PTH increases serum calcium levels by two other mechanisms. PTH increases the synthesis of the active form of vitamin D, 1,25-dihyroxycholecalciferol, in the kidney, which in turn stimulates production of calcium binding protein. Calcium binding protein enhances calcium phosphate absorption from the gut lumen. PTH also inhibits renal calcium excretion, while promoting phosphate excretion, causing a small increase in serum calcium levels.

Sex Hormones

• Androgens

Testosterone

Leydig cells in the testes produce testosterone (smaller amounts produced in ovaries of females) in response to LH stimulation. Testosterone is responsible for male secondary sex characteristics and reproductive capability.

Actions: Enhances development and maintenance of male sex organs, sperm production, muscle mass, libido, and other secondary sex characteristics.

Indications: Androgen deficiency (growth deficits, impotence), delayed puberty in males, palliation of breast cancer, postpartum breast pain and engorgement.

Undesirable Effects: Women – virilism (hirsutism), menstrual irregularities. Men – prostatic hyperplasia or cancer, gynecomastia (high dose or with liver disease), pattern baldness, reduced sperm count (negative feedback). Both sexes – hypercalcemia, coagulopathies, sodium and water retention, hyperlipidemia, atherosclerosis, cholestatic hepatitis, liver cancer.

• Androgen Inhibitor

Finasteride (Proscar®, Propecia®), inhibits conversion of testosterone to 5α-dihydrotestosterone (DHT). It is indicated for benign prostatic hypertrophy and is being tested for prostatic cancer. At lower doses, it is indicated for male pattern baldness.

• Estrogens

Mechanism: Induce transcription of target genes via intracellular receptors (Fig. 10.1).

Indications: Contraception, atrophic vaginitis, osteoporosis, cardiovascular disease associated with menopause, hemorrhagic menstrual bleeding, failure of ovarian development, hirsutism, prostatic cancer.

Undesirable Effects: Nausea (worse in morning, tolerance develops), breast tenderness and edema, and gynecomastia. Increased risk of endometrial cancer.

Contraindications: Pregnancy (teratogenic), estrogen dependent neoplasm, vaginal bleeding, liver impairment, thromboembolic disorders.

Pharmacokinetics: Most estrogens are well absorbed orally. They tend to be rapidly degraded by the liver during their first pass from the gastrointestinal tract. Metabolites include glucuronide and sulfide conjugates of estradiol, estrone, and estriol.

Table 10.1 Testosterone Derivatives

DRUG	UNIQUE PROPERTIES
Testosterone cypionate	IM. Long acting.
Testosterone enanthate	
Testosterone propionate	IM. Short acting. Useful for palliative treatment of breast cancer because therapy can be discontinued rapidly if hypercalcemia develops.
Fluoxymesterone	Short acting oral preparation is more convenient, but less effective than above preparations. Used to treat hypogonadism which develops in adulthood.
Methyltestosterone	Similar to fluoxymesterone. Buccal form available.

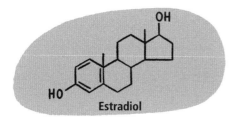
Estradiol

progesterone fails to reach target tissues when administered orally. Synthetic progestins, in contrast, are not susceptible to first pass metabolism and can thus be administered orally.

Progesterone

• Progestins

Mechanism: Induce synthesis of specific proteins via intracellular receptors (Fig. 10.1).

Indications: Contraception, irregular or hemorrhagic menstrual bleeding, endometrial carcinoma, hypoventilation.

Undesirable Effects: Masculinization with prolonged use, otherwise minimal toxicity. Undesirable effects of oral contraceptives described on next page.

Pharmacokinetics: Metabolized by liver to glucuronide or sulfate conjugates. Most of initial dose is rapidly degraded by first pass metabolism, thus

• Oral Contraceptives

Estrogen/Progestin Combinations: Oral contraceptives which contain both estrogen and progestins are the most commonly used form of birth control. They

Table 10.2 Estrogens and Progestins

DRUG	UNIQUE PROPERTIES
Estrogens	
Estradiol (e.g., Estraderm)	Most potent endogenous estrogen secreted by the ovary. Transdermal/IM/PO. Reduces osteoporosis in postmenopausal women. Oral form metabolized to estrone (less active).
17-ethinyl estradiol (e.g., Estinyl)	High potency, not degraded during first pass metabolism (hepatic enzymes fail to recognize this chemically altered estrogen). Used in combination with progestins for contraception.
Conjugated Estrogens (Premarin)	Sulfate esters of estrogenic substances. Less potent than estradiol. Oral, IV, or vaginal preparations are effective.
Progestins	
Progesterone	IM only. Primarily used to treat menstrual disorders.
Medroxyprogesterone (Depo-Provera)	PO/IM. Used for secondary amenorrhea and hormone-induced abnormal uterine bleeding. Intramuscular depot may have prolonged actions. Should be avoided in women who have potential to become pregnant in the near future.
Megestrol (e.g., Megace)	Palliative chemotherapy for breast or endometrial cancer. Also used as an appetite stimulant.
Norethindrone	Potent oral agent.
Estrogen Receptor Modulator	
Raloxifene (Evista)	Binds to estrogen receptor and induces expression of genes that maintain bone density. Indicated for osteoporosis prevention. Is not an estrogen. Does not mimic estrogens in breast or uterus.

are more effective in preventing pregnancy than any other form of contraception and are more convenient than many other forms. Nevertheless, the rate of pregnancy in women using oral contraceptives is higher than would be expected based on careful clinical trials. The most common reason for this is patient failure to take the pill at recommended dosing intervals.

Dosing Regimen: Pills containing active steroids are taken for 21 days of the 28 day cycle. Placebos or iron pills are taken the remaining 7 days to maintain a regimen of one pill per day. During the 7 days of nonsteroid pills, patients experience withdrawal bleeding.

Mechanism of Action: Suppresses ovulation by feedback inhibition at the hypothalamus and pituitary. Estrogen suppresses FSH and progestin suppresses LH. In addition, the steroids directly cause cervical mucosal thickening and render the endometrium "inhospitable" for ovum implantation.

Estrogen Component: ethinyl estradiol or mestranol.

Progestin Component: norethindrone, ethynodiol, norethynodrel, norgestrel, or levonorgestrel.

Dosing Regimen: MONOPHASIC preparations – progestin dose is fixed through the cycle. BIPHASIC and TRIPHASIC contraceptives were created with the intention of more closely mimicking physiologic concentrations of progestins and to decrease side effects by lowering the overall dose of progestins. BIPHASIC pills have low dose progestin for 10 days, followed by 11 days at a higher dose. The concentration of progestin begins low in TRIPHASIC pills, then increases each 7 days through the 21 day cycle. Estrogen concentration is fixed and unchanging in all three formulations. TRIPHASIC pills most closely resemble normal physiology and appear to be as effective as monophasic and biphasic formulations.

Side effects: Improved formulation has dramatically lowered the risk of side effects from birth control pills. Most common side effects are nausea, vomiting, breast tenderness, water retention, and weight gain. Less frequent but more serious side effects include increased risk for thromboembolic episodes, hepatic adenomas, hemorrhagic stroke, myocardial infarction and endometrial cancer. Smoking potentiates risk of myocardial infarction 5-fold in women over 30.

Contraindications: History of thromboembolic disorders, deep venous thrombosis, cerebral vascular disease, myocardial infarction, liver cancer, estrogen-dependent cancer, breast cancer, undiagnosed abnormal genital bleeding, or suspected pregnancy.

Drug Interactions: Contraceptive effects are decreased when taken with ANTIBIOTICS (ampicillin, isoniazid, neomycin, pen V, rifampin, sulfonamides, tetracycline) or CNS AGENTS (barbiturates, benzodiazepines, phenytoin). Contraceptives increase the effects of corticosteroids and worsen side effects of tricyclic antidepressants. Oral contraceptives decrease the effectiveness of oral anticoagulants, anticonvulsants, and oral hypoglycemic agents.

• *Progestin Only "Minipills"*

The mechanism is unclear but they probably act by altering the endometrium to prevent ovum implantation. Minipills are taken every day (there is no 7 day break in the cycle). Missed doses are treated as described for combination products above, except alternate forms of contraception are encouraged for two weeks after omission of two doses. Lack of estrogen may decrease side effects. Continued use may lead to amenorrhea and endometrial atrophy.

• *Levonorgestrel Implants (Norplant®)*

Levonorgestrel implants are synthetic polymer capsules embedded with levonorgestrel, a progestin. The capsules are implanted subcutaneously in women who choose this form of birth control. The capsules continuously release progestin to maintain low contraceptive serum progestin levels. Failure rates are similar to those of oral contraceptives. The most frequent side effects are prolonged, absent, or irregular menstrual bleeding.

Oxytocin and Other OB/GYN Drugs

The posterior pituitary releases two hormones, oxytocin and vasopressin. Oxytocin induces contractions in the gravid uterus and is therefore used when labor acceleration is desired. Because it is chemically similar to vasopressin, oxytocin has antidiuretic effects and can cause fluid retention. Oxytocin, other uterine contractants, and uterine relaxants are listed in Table 10.3.

Obstetricians administer methyl-ergonovine after delivery to reduce uterine hemorrhage. This drug causes vasoconstriction, but more importantly causes tonic uterine contraction. The force of the muscle contraction impedes blood flow through the uterus which significantly reduces bleeding. The other uterine contractants listed in Table 10.3 are used primarily for inducing abortion. Uterine relaxants known as tocolytic agents are β2 adrenergic agonists which reduce contractions in patients with premature onset of labor (Table 10.3).

Three pharmacologic strategies for treating infertility are presented in Table 10.4. Gonadorelin is synthetic GnRH which stimulates FSH and LH production when administered in pulses. Clomiphene is an antiestrogen which causes FSH and LH release by reducing feedback inhibition by estrogen on the pituitary gland. Menotropins are FSH and LH purified from the urine of postmenopausal women. All have greater than 50%

success rate in achieving ovulation and all carry the risk of inducing multiple pregnancies.

Adrenal Hormones

• Glucocorticoids

Cortisol is a glucocorticoid released by the adrenal gland which helps maintain homeostasis by regulating numerous enzymes throughout the body. During periods of stress, cortisol plays an important role in increasing blood glucose levels and elevating blood pressure. Clinically, cortisol and its derivatives are often used for their immunosuppressive properties. They are also important for patients with adrenal deficiencies.

Synthesis: The limbic system ultimately controls cortisone production by regulating release of corticotropin releasing hormone (CRH) from the hypothalamus via serotoninergic, dopaminergic and cholinergic neurons. CRH stimulates release of adrenocorticotrophic hormone (ACTH) from the anterior pituitary. ACTH activates adenylate cyclase in the adrenal cortex. The resulting cAMP activates protein kinase which enhances cholesterol esterase activity. Cholesterol esterase increases the amount of cholesterol available to mitochondria, where cortisone is made from cholesterol. ACTH also stimulates the conversion of cholesterol to pregnenolone, the first step in steroid synthesis.

Transport to tissues: Cortisol is secreted into the blood stream where it is 90% bound to cortisol-binding globulin (CBG) and albumin. Active cortisol (remaining 10%) freely diffuses into cells where it exerts its actions via intracellular receptors. CBG plays an important role in regulating cortisol delivery and clearance. Dexamethasone has low affinity for CBG. It is therefore more potent pharmacologically because a greater fraction is free in the bloodstream.

Metabolism: In the liver, cortisol is converted to dihydro- and tetrahydro- derivatives which are subsequently conjugated with glucuronic acid of sulfates. The conjugates are water soluble and are rapidly excreted by the kidneys. Liver failure leads to decreased metabolism and decreased CBG synthesis. Thus greater amounts of unbound (active) cortisol is present in the blood. This leads to hypercortism. Likewise, renal failure increases the half-life of cortisol.

Clinical Indications: Replacement therapy in adrenocortical insufficiency, salt-losing forms of congenital adrenal hyperplasia, autoimmune diseases, arthritis (Table 10.5), asthma (Table 5.1), dermatitis, cancer (Table 8.5) and sarcoidosis.

Undesirable Effects: Adrenal suppression (insufficiency upon withdrawal), Cushing's Syndrome (osteoporosis, skin atrophy, central fat distribution, abnormal glucose tolerance, behavioral abnormalities), suppression of somatic growth, osteopenia and bone fractures.

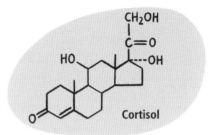

• Adrenocorticosteroid Hypersecretion

Cushing's Syndrome: State of excess glucocorticoids caused by 1) overmedication with drugs listed above, 2) adrenal hypersecretion due to tumor, or 3) excessive ACTH release (pituitary adenoma or metastatic tumors). Results in osteoporosis, skin atrophy, abnormal fat distribution, abnormal glucose tolerance, behavioral abnormalities, euphoria. **Primary Hyperaldosteronism:** Caused by adrenal adenoma which secretes aldosterone. Results in hypertension, hypokalemia, metabolic alkalosis, suppressed renin. **Aminoglutethimide** (Cytadren®) reduces synthesis of adrenal hormones by blocking conversion of cholesterol to Δ^5-pregnenalone.

• Mineralocorticoids & Androgens

The preceding information focused primarily on glucocorticoids. Two other important classes of steroids, mineralocorticoids and androgens, are also produced by the adrenal glands.

Aldosterone is the primary mineralocorticoid. It retains sodium (and subsequently water) in the blood. It is stimulated in the renin-angiotensin pathway.

Dehydroepiandrosterone and androstenedione are the principal androgens. They have little masculinizing effects in men, but are metabolized to testosterone in women, resulting in development of public hair and libido.

Thyroid Hormones

The thyroid gland synthesizes and releases T_3 (3,5,3'-triiodothyronine) and T_4 (thyroxine) which regulate protein synthesis, regulate membrane-bound enzymes and stimulate mitochondrial oxidation. T_3 and T_4 also regulate fetal and infant brain development and childhood growth. T_3 is more potent than T_4.

T_3 and T_4 synthesis: The thyroid follicular cell traps inorganic iodide and oxidizes it to iodine. Iodine binds to tyrosine residues of thyroglobulin to form

Table 10.3 Drugs which Alter Uterine Motility

DRUG	UTERINE ACTIONS	OTHER ACTIONS	INDICATIONS
Uterine Contraction Stimulants			
Oxytocin (e.g., Pitocin)	↑ force and frequency of uterine contractions. Most pronounced in near-term uterus.	Contraction of myoepithelium surrounding alveoli of mammary gland. Antidiuretic (vasopressin) effects.	Drug of choice to induce or accelerate labor, to decrease postpartum uterine bleeding. Stimulates milk ejection from breast (nasal spray).
Ergonovine (Ergotrate Maleate)	Induce uterine smooth muscle contraction.	Blocks adrenergic receptors, causes vasoconstriction, interacts with other receptors (dopamine and tryptamine). ↓ lactation by ↓ prolactin levels.	To ↓ uterine bleeding after abortion or parturition. NOT for induction of labor.
Methyl-ergonovine (Methergine)	" "	" "	" "
Carboprost tromethamine (Prostin/15M)	Synthetic prostaglandin which stimulates uterine contraction.	Regulate smooth muscle tone, coagulation, and body temperature.	Abortion during 2nd trimester.
Dinoprostone (Prostin E2)	" "	" "	Abortion during 2nd trimester. Also used to "ripen" (soften) the cervix prior to induction of labor.
Uterine Relaxants			
Terbutaline (e.g., Bricanyl)	β₂ adrenergic receptor preferring agonist. ↓ uterine smooth muscle contraction in near-term pregnant women.	↑ glycogenolysis, tachycardia, gluconeogenesis, gut relaxation, and vasodilation. ↓ respiration of mast cells and neutrophils.	Prolong gestation in premature labor cases.
Ritodrine	" "	" "	" "
Magnesium	Decreases uterine contraction.	Decreases neuromuscular conduction, ↓ acetylcholine release, vasodilation, respiratory depression at high doses.	Premature onset of labor, pre-eclampsia, eclampsia.

Table 10.4 Drugs Used to Treat Infertility

DRUG	SUMMARY
Gonadorelin	Gonadrenalin is synthetic human gonadotropin-releasing hormone (GnRH). Gonadorelin is administered intravenously in pulses spaced 90 minutes apart. Like endogenous GnRH, the pulses of gonadrenalin stimulate FSH and LH release and result in ovulation in about 90% of women who have been treated. The rate of multiple pregnancies was 12% in a small series. When administered continuously, rather than in pulses, GnRH analogs (Lupron®) suppress FSH and LH production by acting as feedback inhibitors. Administered in this fashion, GnRH analogs are approved for the treatment of prostate cancer and endometriosis.
Clomiphene (e.g., Clomid)	Clomiphene stimulates LH and FSH release by reducing negative-feedback by estrogen on the pituitary. Increased LH and FSH levels induces ovulation and maintains functional corpus lutea. The rate of multiple pregnancies is 8%. Abnormal ovarian enlargement occurs in 14% of patients and may cause pain.
Menotropins (Pergonol)	Menotropins are LH and FSH (purified from urine of postmenopausal women) which are administered intramuscularly for 9–12 days and followed by an injection of chorionic gonadotropin. Multiple births occur in 20% of menotropin-induced pregnancies. Ovarian hyperstimulation, hemoperitoneum, febrile reactions and arterial thromboembolism are the most frequent undesirable effects.

PHARMACOKINETICS	UNDESIRABLE EFFECTS	DRUG INTERACTIONS	NOTES
IV/IM/nasal. Short half-life (3–5 min.).	Potential for uterine tetany or rupture, trauma to infant, post-delivery uterine atony. Prolonged infusion (>24 h) may cause water intoxication (antidiuretic activity).	Potentiates hypertensive effects of other drugs. May cause stroke/hemorrhage, fetal distress.	Synthetic oxytocin mimics the effects of endogenous oxytocin which is released from the hypothalamus.
	Hypertension. May cause death of infant if given prior to delivery. Potentially fatal poisoning may occur at normal doses in patients sensitive to ergot alkaloids.	" "	
" "	" "	" "	" "
IM. Short half-life. Mean time to abortion is 16 hours.	Incomplete abortion. Nausea, vomiting, fever. Uterine rupture, perforation, inflammation, cramps, CNS, cardiovascular and respiratory complications.	" "	20% saline solution is preferred for abortion. Consider alternatives for women with previous C-sections.
PO/IM/IV/amniotically. Mean time to abortion is 10–15 hours.	" "	" "	" "
IV/PO. Crosses placenta.	Hypotension, tachycardia (reflex and β1 stimulated), arrhythmia, pulmonary edema. Bradycardia, w/abrupt withdrawal. Nausea, headache, muscle tremor.	Corticosteroids ↑ diabetogenic effects. Inhalation anesthetics ↑ hypotension.	
IV/PO.	Similar to terbutaline. More severe hypotension/tachycardia.	" "	
IM/IV. If IM, onset = 1 hr, duration = 3.5 hrs. If IV, onset = seconds, duration = 30 min.	>8 mEq/L may cause depression of CNS, heart and reflexes. Flushing, sweating, hypotension and flaccid paralysis may occur.	Additive with CNS depressants, potentiates neuromuscular blockers, ↑ toxicity of digitalis.	Excess Ca^{++} antagonizes Mg^{++} and is used to counteract CNS and PNS depression.

Table 10.5 Actions of Glucocorticoids

(Generally: anabolic in liver (gluconeogenesis) and catabolic in muscle, skin, lymph, adipose, and connective tissue)

Protein Metabolism:	Carbohydrate Metabolism:	Fat distribution:
↑ catabolism ↓ anabolism	↑ gluconeogenesis ↓ insulin binding to receptors	Redistribute fat toward truncal obesity
Electrolytes:	Immune System:	Blood cytology:
↑ sodium retention ↑ potassium excretion metabolic alkalosis ↓ GI calcium absorption	↓ antibody production ↓ inflammatory reaction ↓ immunocompetent lymphocytes ↓ antigen processing	↑ erythropoesis ↑ neutrophils ↓ lymphocytes
Water:	Brain:	Gastrointestinal tract:
↑ free water clearance	↓ threshold for electrical excitation	↑ acid and pepsin secretion thinning of mucus

Table 10.6 Cortisone Derivatives

CORTICOSTEROID	IMPORTANT PROPERTIES
Hydrocortisone (Solu-cortef)	PO/IV/IM/Top. Chemically identical to cortisol produced by adrenal glands. Preferred drug for replacement therapy. Has weak mineralocorticoid effects. Short acting.
Prednisone	PO. Intermediate duration of action. Compared to hydrocortisone, glucocorticoid effects are four times more potent and mineralocorticoid effects are half as potent. Drug of choice for maintenance therapy of severe asthma. Important agent in leukemia therapy.
Prednisolone	PO/IV/IM. Intermediate duration of action. Compared to hydrocortisone, glucocorticoid effects are five times more potent and mineralocorticoid effects are half as potent. Drug of choice for treatment of acute asthmatic attacks (administered intravenously for this indication).
Triamcinolone (e.g., Aristocort)	PO/IV/Top/Inh. Intermediate duration of action. Compared to hydrocortisone, glucocorticoid effects are thirty times more potent. No mineralocorticoid effects.
Dexamethasone (Decadron)	PO/IV/IM/Inh. In addition to uses listed in text, it is used to reduce elevated intracranial pressure. Few mineralocorticoid effects. **Dexamethasone suppression test** examines whether the hypothalamus/pituitary can be suppressed by glucocorticoids. If the plasma cortisol level is <5 μg/dl eight hours after receiving 1 gm of dexamethasone, Cushing's syndrome is ruled out.
Fludrocortisone (e.g., Florinef)	PO. Halogenated derivative with potent mineralocorticoid effects. Only oral mineralocorticoid replacement available. Inappropriate for use as an antiinflammatory agent.

Table 10.7 Inhibitors of Adrenal Hormone Synthesis and Actions

DRUG	MECHANISM/ACTIONS	NOTES
Mitotane (Lysodren)	Destroys adrenocortical cells.	Used for palliative treatment of metastatic adrenal carcinoma.
Metyrapone (Metopirone)	Blocks 11B-hydroxylase activity, thus inhibiting steroid synthesis.	Under investigation for use in Cushing's disease.
Aminoglutethamide (Cytadren)	Blocks conversion of cholesterol to Δ^5-pregnenolone (the first step in steroid synthesis).	Uses: Cushing's disease; adjunct to irradiation in preparing patients for adrenalectomy; treatment of adrenal, breast, and ACTH-producing tumors.
Cyproheptadine (Periactin)	Serotonin and cholinergic antagonist which may inhibit secretion of ACTH from pituitary microadenoma cells.	Experimental agent for treatment of ACTH hypersecretion and Cushing's disease.
Spironolactone (Aldactone)	Antagonist of aldosterone, inhibits Na^+ retention.	Treatment of hyperaldosteronism. Causes K^+ retention. Diuretic actions are described in Table 4.3A.

monoiodotyrosine (MIT) and diiodotyrosine (DIT). Then, either two DIT molecules couple to form T_4, or MIT couples with DIT, forming T_3 (Fig. 10.2). T_4 production exceeds T_3 production in the thyroid gland and T_4 is converted to T_3 in the periphery.

T_3 and T_4 release and transport: Thyroglobulin is proteolyzed from T_3 and T_4 and the hormones are released into the circulation. Only 20% of circulating T_3 is secreted by the thyroid. The remainder is derived from degradation of T_4. **Thyroxine-binding globulin** (TBG) and prealbumin carry most T_3 and T_4 molecules in the blood, protecting the hormones from degradation. Only free (unbound) T_3 and T_4 are physiologically active. Feedback mechanisms at the hypothalamus, pituitary gland and thyroid gland inhibit or stimulate T_3 and T_4 production when free thyroid hormone levels are too high or too low, respectively.

• Hyperthyroidism (thyrotoxicosis)

Clinical Features: Nervousness, weakness, heat intolerance, sweating, weight loss, warm thin skin, exophthalmos, loose stool. Known as Grave's disease when goiter and ocular signs are present.

Etiology: Thyroid-stimulating antibodies bind to TSH receptors, causing release of thyroxin (current theory).

Lab Findings: Increased serum T_4 and T_3 levels and increased radioiodide uptake.

Therapeutic Strategy: Control hyperthyroidism with drugs (propylthiouracil or methimazole) for one year, then, partial resection of thyroid gland.

Thyroid Storm: Observed in hyperthyroid patients at the time of thyroidectomy (surgical trauma causes instantaneous release of thyroid hormones) or in hyperthyroid patients in sepsis. Signs include high fever, irritability, delerium, tachycardia, vomiting, diarrhea and hypotension. Coma may develop. Treatment includes IV glucose and saline, vitamin B, glucocorticoids.

• Hypothyroidism

Clinical Features: Fatigue, weakness, cold intolerance, hoarseness, constipation, cold dough-like skin, thick tongue, bradycardia, excessive menstrual bleeding, anemia. Cretinism in childhood.

Etiology: 1) Primary hypothyroidism - surgery, radioiodine ablation, thyroiditis. 2) Secondary hypothyroidism - hypofunction of pituitary or hypothalamus.

Lab Findings: Hypothyroid patients have low concentrations of T_4 in their serum. The uptake of radioactive iodide is low because thyroid stores of iodine are not being used to produce thyroid hormones. The pituitary hormone, thyroid-stimulating hormone (TSH), is high in primary hypothyroidism and low in secondary hypothyroidism.

Therapeutic Strategy: Replacement therapy with purified or synthetic thyroid hormones (Table 10.8).

Myxedema Coma: Chronic, severe hypothyroidism results in respiratory depression, hypothermia and stupor. It is frequently fatal.

Pancreatic Hormones

Insulin is produced by pancreatic islet beta cells and is released in response to elevated serum glucose concentrations. The principle actions of insulin are presented in Table 10.9. Each of these actions reduces the plasma glucose concentration.

• Diabetes Mellitus

Insulin-dependent diabetes mellitus (IDDM: Type 1) is due to an absolute deficiency of insulin which usually develops by age 15 and results in weight loss, hyperglycemia, ketoacidosis, atherosclerosis, retinal damage and kidney failure. Because the pancreatic

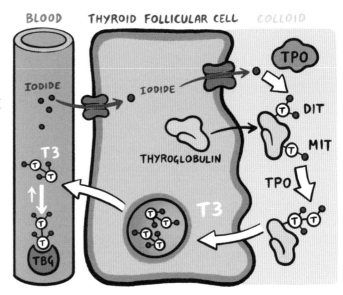

Figure 10.2 Synthesis of T_3. *Schematic drawing of T_3 synthesis as described in the text. T_3 is formed by the coupling of one diiodinated and one monoiodinated tyrosine on thyroglobulin. T_4 synthesis follows the same pathways shown in the figure except that two diiodinated tyrosine molecules couple to form T_4.* **Abbreviations:** *DIT – diiodinated tyrosine, MIT – monoiodinated tyrosine, T3 – 3,5,3'-triiodothyronine, TBG – thyroxin-binding globulin, TPO - thyroid peroxidase.*

islet beta cells (which produce insulin) are damaged or destroyed, oral hypoglycemics cannot induce insulin release. Thus, patients require insulin injections.

Noninsulin-dependent diabetes mellitus (NIDDM: Type II) is due to decreased release of insulin or decreased response of tissue to insulin (e.g., decreased number of insulin receptors) resulting in hyperglycemia but not ketoacidosis. Treatment focuses on diet and exercise, oral hypoglycemic drugs if diet fails, and insulin when all else fails.

• Insulin Replacement

Patients with insulin-dependent diabetes receive subcutaneous insulin injections daily. The goal of insulin therapy is to provide adequate glucose control through each 24 hour period while minimizing the number of injections required to achieve that control. Repeated injections at the same site may result in atrophy or hyperplasia at the injection site. Insulin preparations of short, intermediate and long duration are available (Table 10.10).

Human insulin (Humulin) is prepared by recombinant DNA technology or is synthesized from porcine insulin (enzymatic replacement of the terminal arginine with threonine). Human insulin is preferred to insulin prepared from animals because it is less antigenic. Porcine insulin differs from human insulin by one amino acid (terminal arginine). Bovine insulin is the most immunogenic preparation. A typical dosing regimen con-

Table 10.8 Drugs Used to Treat Thyroid Disorders

DRUG	MECHANISM/ACTIONS	INDICATIONS	UNDESIRABLE EFFECTS
Drugs Used to Treat Hyperthyroidism			
Methimazole (Tapazole)	Inhibits transformation of inorganic iodine to organic iodine. Thyroxine can't be formed without organic iodine. Also inhibits iodotyrosine coupling. No clinical effects observed for several days.	Control hyperthyroidism until surgery or[131]I therapy. Long term drug treatment to avoid surgery or[131]I therapy. About half of patients will remain euthyroid if drug is withdrawn after prolonged use.	Temporary hypothyroidism (treat with thyroxine), agranulocytosis, rash, hyperplastic thyroid. Not given to women who are likely to become pregnant within 3 years. Damages thyroid of fetus.
Propylthiouracil (PTU)	" " Also, blocks conversion of T_4 to T_3 in peripheral tissues.	" "	" "
Iodine/iodide	Inhibits release of thyroxine from thyroid gland. Effects are faster (1–3 days) but weaker than methimazole or PTU. Useful for two weeks, then gland adapts and resumes thyroxine secretion.	Adjunctive therapy used in conjunction with drugs listed above. Provides more rapid relief in severely ill patients. Used to devascularize thyroid gland prior to thyroidectomy.	Folliculitis, fever.
Drug which relieves symptoms of hyperthyroidism			
Propranolol (Inderal)	β adrenergic receptor antagonist. Suppresses tachycardia and other catecholamine effects.	Emergent preparation of hyperthyroid patients for surgery. Thyrotoxicosis in pregnancy. Thyroid storm.	CNS sedation and depression. Suppression of failing heart.
Drugs Used to Treat Hypothyroidism			
Levothyroxine (T4) (Synthroid, Levothroid)	Replaces normal serum levels of T_4 and T_3 (T_4 is converted into T3 by deiodination in the periphery).	Drug of choice for hypothyroidism.	No toxicity at replacement concentration. Overdose causes hyperthyroid effects (top of page).
Liothyronine (T3) (Cytomel)	Replaces T_3.	Used in hypothyroid patients who have difficulty absorbing lovothyroxino.	" "
Liotrix (T4 & T3)	Replaces T_4 and T_3	When conversion of T_4 to T_3 is abnormally low (myxedema coma), liotrix may be more useful than levothyroxine.	" "

Table 10.9 Actions of insulin

SITE	ACTIONS
Muscle	↑ glucose transport into cell ↑ glycogenesis ↑ protein and triglyceride synthesis
Liver	↑ glucose transport into cell ↑ glycogenesis ↑ glucose utilization in Krebs cycle ↑ protein synthesis
Adipose	↑ glucose transport into cell ↑ glycogenesis ↑ triglyceride synthesis

sists of regular humulin with either lente or NPH two to three times per day before meals.

Insulin Toxicity: The most common undesirable effects of insulin administration are hypoglycemia and hypokalemia. Hypoglycemia is manifested by weakness, hunger, sweating, dizziness, tachycardia, anxiety, tremor, headaches, mental disturbances and visual disturbances. Many of these symptoms are caused by hypoglycemic release of epinephrine (epinephrine causes glycogenolysis, gluconeogenesis and lipolysis and inhibits insulin release). Remaining symptoms are due to the brain being starved of its energy supply.

Hypokalemia develops because insulin drives potassium from serum into cells. It is most often

Table 10.10 Insulin Preparations

DRUG	ONSET (HRS)	DURATION (HRS)	TRADE NAMES
Rapid-Acting			
Regular Insulin	0.5–1	5–8	Humulin R, Novolin R, Regular Iletin II, Velosulin.
Prompt Insulin Zinc Suspension	1–2	12–16	
Lispro Insulin Solution	0.25	6–8	Humalog, Admelog, Basaglar
Insulin glulisine	0.5–1.5	1–2.5	Apidra
Intermediate Acting			
Isophane Insulin Suspension	1–2	24–28	Humulin N, Novolin N.
Insulin Zinc Suspension	1–3	24–28	Humulin L, Lente Insulin, Lente Iletin I and II, Novolin L.
Insulin glargine	1	24	Lantus, Toujeo
Long Acting			
Extended Insulin Zinc Suspension	4–8	>36	Humulin U Ultralente.
Insulin degludec (ultra-long)	0.5–1.5	>42	Tresiba
Combination Product			
Isophane Insulin Suspension and Insulin Injection	0.25–1	24	Novolin 70/30, Humulin 70/30 Humulin 50/50

encountered in patients with ketoacidosis when insulin therapy is instituted. Severe hypokalemia causes cardiac arrhythmias and neuromuscular disturbances. Repeated injections at the same site may result in atrophy or hyperplasia at the injection site.

• *Oral Hypoglycemic Drugs*

Patients with noninsulin-dependent diabetes mellitus (Type 2) who fail dietary control require oral hypoglycemic agents. The sulfonylureas described in Table 10.11 stimulate insulin secretion by pancreatic beta cells and increase the sensitivity of tissues to the actions of insulin. Like insulin, the most frequent complication is hypoglycemia. Newer generations of oral hypoglycemics reduce post-prandial sugar levels or increase the sensitivity of target tissues to insulin. Nonsulfonylureas are less likely to cause hypoglycemia. Because diabetes damages kidneys and livers, dose adjustments may be necessary. Patients with NIDDM who fail dietary control and oral hypoglycemic agents progress to insulin-dependency.

Anti-Obesity and Appetite Suppression Drugs

Glucagon-like peptide-1 (GLP-1) is a hormone produced by your body that causes insulin release, suppresses appetite, and makes individuals feel full longer. GLP-1 agonists (**semaglutide** (Wegovy) and **liraglutide** (Saxenda) are approved to treat obesity in adults with a body mass index (BMI) of 30 kg/m^2 or higher and liragluitide is also approved in adolescents with obesity. Liraglutide is administered by self-injection daily and semaglutide is injected once weekly. Semaglutide was more effective than liraglutide in terms of weight loss in a comparison trial. These and other GLP-1 agonists are used to treat type 2 diabetes (see full list in Table 10.11). Both drugs cause nausea in about 40% of subjects and each causes other gastrointestinal side effects less commonly. Both can cause thyroid C-cell tumors in mice, but this risk has not been confirmed in humans. Pancreatitis, hypoglycemia, gallbladder dysfunction, tachycardia, and suicidal thoughts have been reported and are not common. Caution should be used in patients who take insulin or insulin-releasing medicines (e.g., sulfonylureas).

Another medication approved for obesity is **orlistat** (Xenical) which inhibits lipase, an enzyme released by the pancreas that breaks down fats so they can be easily absorbed. Combinations of phentermine-topiramate (Qsimia) and naltrexone-bupriopion (Contrave) are also approved for obesity management. Medications approved for short-term (<12 weeks) appetite suppression include **phentermine, benzphetamine, diethylpropion, and phendimetrazine.**

Table 10.11 Anti-hyperglycemic (glucose lowering) drugs

DRUG	NOTES
Oral Hypoglycemics: Sulfonylureas	
Tolbutamide (Orinase) **Tolazamide** (Tolinase) **Chlorpropamide** (Diabinese) **Glipizide** (Glucotrol) **Glyburide** (Micronase, Diabeta) **Glimepiride** (Amaryl)	Stimulates insulin secretion by pancreatic beta cells and increases the sensitivity of tissues to the actions of insulin. May cause hypoglycemia. Patients who develop hypoglycemia while taking **Chlorpropamide** must be monitored carefully for 3–5 days because of its long half-life (60–90 hours). Clinical trials revealed unexpected increased risk of cardiotoxicity when **Tolbutamide** was used for more than five years.
Oral Hypoglycemics: Nonsulfonylureas	
Metformin (Glucophage)	Reduces intestinal uptake and hepatic production of glucose. Increases sensitivity of tissues to insulin. Generally does not cause hypoglycemia. May act synergistically with sulfonylureas. Rarely causes lactic acidosis, which is potentially fatal (see warnings). More commonly causes gastrointestinal side effects.
Miglitol (Glyset) **Acarbose** (Precose)	Alpha glucoside inhibitor slows carbohydrate digestion resulting in lower serum glucose levels after meals. May be used with sulfonylureas. Hypoglycemia unlikely when used as a single agent. Flatulance, diarrhea and abdominal pain are the most frequent side effects.
Rosiglitazone (Avandia) **Pioglitazone** (Actos)	Enhances response of target cells (e.g., liver, muscle) to endogenous insulin, perhaps by activating nuclear receptors that increase transcription of glucose control genes. Because these require endogenous insulin, they should not be used for Type I diabetes or diabetic ketoacidosis. Monitor liver function tests (LFTs). Discontinue drug if LFTs are greater than 3-times normal. May increase incidence of congestive heart failure and MI.
Repaglinide (Prandin)	Blocks potassium channels in pancreatic beta cells, causing depolarization, calcium influx, and ultimately insulin secretion. Thus reduces glucose levels through mechanism that requires intact beta cells. Used alone or with metformin for type 2 diabetes that is diet refractory.
Nateglinide (Starlix)	Stimulates insulin secretion from pancreas.
Dapagliflozin (Farxiga) **Canagliflozin** (Invokana) **Empagliflozin** (Jardiance)	Inhibits sodium-glucose transporter 2 (SGLT2), which reduces the amount of sugar absorbed by the body. Used for type II diabetes along with diet and exercise.
Peptides that mimic glucagon-like peptide-1 (GLP-1) or amylin	
Liraglutide (Victoza) **Exenatide** (Bydureon) **Dulaglutide** (Trulicity) **Albiglutide** (Tanzeum) **Lixisenatide** (Lyxumia, Adlyxin) **Semaglutide** (Ozempic, Wegovy)	These peptide drugs are administered subcutaneously. They mimic natural peptides called "Incretins" that increase insulin levels. Long-acting analog of glucagon-like peptide -1 (GLP-1), which increases the amount of insulin that the body produces. Used for type II diabetes along with diet and exercise. Some of these agents cause thyroid cancer in mice and it is not yet known whether they increase the risk of cancer in humans. Some are available in fixed-dose combination with insulin.
Pramlintide (Symlin Pen)	This is an injectable medicine that slows digestion of food, which prevents blood sugar from rising rapidly after eating. It is used in conjunction with insulin and may cause hypoglycemia when used in combination.
Dipeptidyl peptidase IV (DPP-4) inhibitors and sodium glucose transporter 2 (SGL-2) inhibitors	
Saxagliptin (Onglyza) **Sitagliptin** (Steglujan) **Linagliptin** (Tradjenta) **Alogliptin** (Vipidia)	Oral medications that inhibit DPP-4, the enzyme that helps break down incretin hormones (e.g., GLP-1 (see above) and glucose-dependent insulinotropic polypeptide (GIP)). GLP-1 and GIP are produced by the intestine, with increased amounts released after meals. By blocking DPP-4, GLP-1 and GIP levels are increased and this leads to increased insulin production when glucose levels are normal or high.
Ertugliflozin (Steglatro) **Bexaglifozin** (Brenzavvy)	Oral medicine that inhibit SGLT2, which is a transporter that reabsorbs glucose from glomerular filtrate so that it re-enters the bloodstream. Should not be used in patients with renal failure.
Combinations	
Ertugliflozin/Sitagliptin (Steglujan) **Ertugliflozin/Metformin** (Segluromet) **Dapagliflozin/Saxagliptin** (Qtern) **Empaglifozin/Metformin** (Synjardy) **Empaglifozin/linagliptin** (Glyxambi)	

Helpful Hint Regarding Drug Names:

-tide: Drugs with names that end in "tide" are peptides. Because peptides are typically not absorbed by the gut, they are not typically administered orally. Because most peptides are small enough to pass through glomeruli in the kidney, they typically have a very short half-life. For these reasons, many peptide drugs are administered subcutaneously. If the peptide has a net positive charge, it may interact with negatively charged glycoproteins in subcutaneous fat, which results in slow release from fat (a depot effect) which helps reduce the need for frequent dosing.

INDEX

Hydrocortisone, 156
Hydromorphone, 48
Hydroxy-amphetamine, 18
Hydroxychloroquine, 141
Hydroxyurea, 130
Hydroxyzine, 146
Hylorel, 20, 64
Hypoglycemics, 160
Hytrin, 74

I
Ibalizumab, 118
Ibrance, 130
Ibritumomab, 135
Ibrutinib, 133
Ibuprofen, 84, 140
Ibutilide, 80
Iclusig, 131
Idarubicin, 128
Ifosfamide, 126
Ilex, 126
Iloperidone, 44
Ilumya, 142
Imatinib, 131
Imbruvica, 133
Imfinzi, 134
Imipenem, 104
Imipramine, 36
Imitrex®, 55
Imjudo, 134
Immunostimulants, 139, 144
Immunosuppressants, 139, 144
Imodium, 96
Imuran, 144
Incruse, 88
Indacaterol, 88
Inderal, 22, 66, 80, 158
Indocin, 140
Indomethacin, 140
Infigratinib, 132
Infliximab, 141
Ingrezza, 49
Inlyta, 131
Inotuzumab Ozogamicin, 134
Inrebic, 132
Inspra, 68
Insulin, 10, 159
Insulin Degludec, 159
Insulin Glargine, 159
Insulin Glulisine, 159
Insulin Zinc Suspension, 159
Intal, 90
Integrilin, 84
Intelence, 118
Interferon, 135
Interferon Beta-1, 143
Interferons, 144
Interleukin II, 137
Intropin, 16
Invanz, 104
Invega Sustenna, 44
Invokana, 160
Iodide, 158
Iodine, 158
Ipilimumab, 134
Ipratropium, 88

Irbesartan, 68
Iressa, 131
Irinotecan, 129
Isatuximab, 135
Isentress, 118
Ismelin, 20
Isocaine, 32
Isocarboxazid, 36
Isoflurane, 58
Isoniazid, 115
Isophane Insulin Suspension, 159
Isoproterenol, 16, 88
Isopten, 70
Isopto Carbachol, 24
Isopto-Carpine, 24
Isordil, 71
Isosorbide Dinitrate, 71
Isotretinoin, 130
Isoxsuprine, 68
Isradipine, 70
Istodax, 130
Isuprel, 16, 88
Itraconazole, 120
Ivabradine, 74
Ivermectin, 122
Ivosidenib, 130
Ixabepilone, 129
Ixazomib, 130
Ixekizumab, 142
Ixempra, 129

J
Jakafi, 132
Jardiance, 160
Jaypirca, 133
Jempesli, 134
Jevtana, 129
Juxtapid, 82

K
Kanamycin, 112, 115
Kaolin/Pectin, 96
Kaopectate, 96
Keflex, 108
Kefzol, 108
Kemadrin, 28
Keppra, 56
Kerlone, 22, 66, 80
Kesimpta, 143
Ketalar, 58
Ketamine, 58
Ketek, 112
Ketolides, 112
Ketoprofen, 140
Ketorolac, 10, 140
Kevzara, 141
Keytruda, 134
Kimmtrak, 135
Kineret, 141
Kisquali, 130
Klonopin, 54
Koselugo, 132
Krystexxa, 142
Kwell, 122
Kyprolis, 130
Kytril, 45

L
Labetalol, 22, 66
Lacosamide, 56
Lactulose, 98
Lamictal, 56
Lamivudine, 117, 118
Lamotrigine, 56
Lanoxin, 74, 80
Lansoprazole, 94
Lantus, 159
Lapatinib, 131, 133
Larotrectinib, 133
Lartruvo, 132
Lasix, 62
Latuda, 42
Laxative, 12
Laxatives, 98
Lecanemab, 50
Ledipasvir, 117
Leflunomide, 141
Lenacapavir, 118
Lenalidomide, 135
Lente Iletin I, 159
Lente Iletin II, 159
Lente Insulin, 159
Lenvatinib, 131
Lenvima, 131
Leqembi, 49
Lescol, 82
Lesinurad, 142
Leukeran, 126
Leukine, 137
Leuprolide, 136
Leustatin, 127
Levalbuteral, 88
Levalbuterol, 16
Levamisole, 144
Levaquin, 110
Levatol, 22, 66
Levetiracetam, 56
Levo-dromoran, 48
Levocetirizine, 146
Levodopa, 46
Levofloxacin, 110
Levomilnacipran, 38
Levonorgesterel Implant, 152
Levophed, 16
Levorphanol, 48
Levothroid, 158
Levothyroxine T4, 158
Lexapro, 38
Lexiva, 118
Librium, 54
Libtayo, 134
Lidocaine, 32, 78
Linagliptin, 160
Lincocin, 112
Lincomycin, 112
Lincosamides, 112
Lindane, 122
Linezolid, 112
Liothyronine T3, 158
Liotrix T4 & T3, 158
Lipitor, 82
Lipopeptides, 104
Liraglutide, 160

Nicardipine, 70
Nicotine, 24–25
Nifedipine, 60, 70
Nimbex, 30
Ninlaro, 130
Nintedanib, 132
Nipride, 68
Niraparib, 130
Nisoldipine, 70
Nitrofurantoin, 110
Nitroglycerin, 60, 61, 71
Nitroprusside, 61, 68
Nitrous Oxide, 58
Nivolumab, 134
Nizatidine, 94, 146
Norcuron, 30
Norepinephrine, 16, 34
Norethindrone, 151
Norfloxacin, 110
Normodyne, 22
Noroxin, 110
Norpace, 78
Norplant®, 152
Norpramin, 36
Nortriptyline, 36
Norvasc, 70
Norvir, 118
Novantrone, 128, 143
Novocaine, 32
Novolin 70/30, 159
Novolin L, 159
Novolin N, 159
Novolin R, 159
Noxafil, 120
NSAIDS, 140, 141, 142, 144
Nucala, 90
Nuplazid, 42
Nuromax, 30
Nurtec, 55
Nuvigil, 40
Nystatin, 120

O
Obinutuzumab, 135
Ocrelizumab, 135, 143
Ocrevus, 135, 143
Odomzo, 130
Ofatumumab, 135, 143
Ofev, 132
Ofloxacin, 110
Olanzapine, 44
Olaparib, 130
Olaratumab, 132
Olmesartan, 68
Olodaterol, 88
Olsalazine, 96, 140
Olumiant, 141
Omadacycline, 112
Omalizumab, 92
Ombitasvir, 117
Omeprazole, 94
Omnaris, 92
Oncovin, 129
Ondansetron, 45
Onglyza, 160
Onzetra Xsail, 55

Opdivo, 134
Opiod, 35
Oprelvekin, 137
Orap, 44
Orencia, 141
Oretic, 62
Orinase, 160
Oritavancin, 104
Oseltamivir, 116
Osimertinib, 131
Osmotic Diuretics, 62
Oxacillin, 106
Oxaliplatin, 129
Oxazepam, 54
Oxybate, 40
Oxybutynin, 28
Oxycarbazepine, 56
Oxycodone, 48
Oxycontin, 48
Oxymorphone, 48
Oxytetracycline, 112
Oxytocin, 154
Ozanimod, 143
Ozempic, 160

P
Paclitaxel, 129
Pacritinib, 132
Padcev, 134
Palanosetron, 45
Palbociclib, 130
Palilperidone, 44
Palivizumab, 92
Pamelor, 36
Pamine, 28
Pancuronium, 30
Panitumumab, 131
Pantoprazole, 94
Papaverine, 68
Para-aminosalicylic Acid, 115
Paractant, 92
Paraplatin, 129
Parcopa, 46
Paritaprevir, 117
Parlodel, 46
Parnate, 36
Paroxetine, 38
Pavabid, 68
Pavulon, 30
Paxil, 38
Pazopanib, 131
Pegasys, 117
PegInterferon, 117
Peginterferon Beta-1A, 143
Pegloticase, 142
Pemaglitinib, 132
Pemazyre, 132
Pembrolizumab, 134
Penbutolol, 22, 66
Penciclovir, 116
Penicillin G, 106
Penicillin V, 106
Penicillins, 104, 106
Pentam, 119
Pentamidine, 119
Pentobarbital, 54

Pentothal, 58
Pepcid, 94, 146
Pepto-Bismol, 96
Perampanel, 56
Perforomist, 88
Pergonol, 154
Periactin, 156
Perindopril, 67
Perjeta, 133
Perphenazine, 42
Persantine, 84
Pertuzumab, 133
Pexadartinib, 132
Phenelzine, 36
Phenergan, 45, 146
Phenobarbital, 53, 54
Phenoxybenzamine, 22
Phentolamine, 22
Phenylephrine, 16
Phenytoin, 53, 56
Phospholine Iodide, 26
Physostigmine, 26
Pifeltro, 118
Pilocar, 24
Pilocarpine, 24
Pimavanserin, 42
Pimozide, 44
Pindolol, 22, 66
Pioglitazone, 160
Piperacillin, 106
Piqray, 133
Pirbuterol, 16, 88
Piroxicam, 140
Pirtobrutinib, 133
Pitavastatin, 82
Pitocin, 154
Pitolisant, 40
Plaquenil, 122
Platinol-AQ, 129
Plavix, 84
Plazomicin, 112
Plecanatide, 98
Plegridy, 143
Plendil, 70
Pletal, 84
Polaramine, 146
Polatuzumab Vedotin, 134
Polivy, 134
Polocaine, 32
Polyenes, 120
Polyethylene Glycol, 98
Pomalidomide, 135
Pomalyst, 135
Ponatinib, 131
Ponesimod, 143
Ponstel, 140
Pontocaine, 32
Ponvory, 143
Portrazza, 131
Posaconazole, 120
Potassium Sparing Diuretics, 62
Poteligeo, 135
Pradaxa, 84
Pralsetinib, 132
Praluent, 82
Pramipexole, 46